THE INFERTILITY MAZE

Finding Your Way to the Right Help and the Right Answers

KASSIE SCHWAN

CB
CONTEMPORARY
BOOKS
CHICAGO · NEW YORK

Library of Congress Cataloging-in-Publication Data

Schwan, Kassie.
    The infertility maze : finding your way to the right help and the right answers. / Kassie Schwan.
       p.   cm.
    Bibliography: p.
    ISBN 0-8092-4534-5
    1. Infertility—Popular works.   I. Title.
RC889.S35   1988
616.6'92—dc19   88-28130
                                                                          CIP

Copyright © 1988 by Kassie Schwan
All rights reserved
Published by Contemporary Books, Inc.
180 North Michigan Avenue, Chicago, Illinois 60601
Manufactured in the United States of America
International Standard Book Number: 0-8092-4534-5

Published simultaneously in Canada by Beaverbooks, Ltd.
195 Allstate Parkway, Valleywood Business Park
Markham, Ontario L3R 4T8 Canada

For Brian

The information contained in this book is for educational purposes only. Only your physician can determine what tests and treatments are best for you.

Contents

Acknowledgments	ix
Foreword by Dr. Sherman Silber	xi
Introduction: What Is the Infertility Maze?	1

SECTION I
WHEN YOU REALIZE YOU HAVE A PROBLEM

Introduction to Section I	8
Are You Worried That You Might Not Be Able to Have a Baby?	9
The Questions You Worry About	9
ESSAY: *A Future Without Children*	19
Does Worrying Affect Fertility? Should You Just "Relax"?	21
"Adopt, and You'll Get Pregnant."	22
Do You Need a Specialist Yet?	23
How to Find and Choose a Specialist	27
Learning About Reproduction, Fertility and Infertility	29
Home Remedies for Infertility	31
Reviewing Your Medical History	33
Notes for Female Medical History	34
Notes for Male Medical History	36
Start Your Temperature Charts	38
ESSAY: *Thoughts About Taking Your Temperature*	43
Using Urine Testing Kits to Watch for Ovulation	44
Watching for Changes in Cervical Mucus	45
Making Love by the Calendar	46

SECTION II
YOUR INFERTILITY IS INVESTIGATED: THE WORKUPS

Introduction to Section II	50
As Your Appointment Approaches, How Are You Feeling?	51
Talking Together About Your Expectations	53
The First Appointment: How to Evaluate Your Specialist	53
Questions to Ask the Specialist at the First Appointment	55
Talking to Your Doctor	56
The Workup is Planned	57

Overview of the Workup: Women	59
Overview of the Workup: Men	62
Coping with the Inconveniences of the Workups	63
Coping With Infertility: Your Methods May Differ	66
The Woman's Workup	68
Notes on the Physical and Pelvic Exam	73
Notes on BBT's	74
Record of Postcoital Examinations	75
ESSAY: *Your Cervical Mucus is Gorgeous*	77
ESSAY: *The Instructions Are Simple Enough*	78
Record of Hysterosalpingogram	82
ESSAY: *I've Been on Both Sides of the X-Ray Equipment*	83
Record of your Endometrial Biopsy	86
ESSAY: *My Endometrial Biopsy*	87
Record of Diagnostic Laparoscopy	91
ESSAY: *A Laparoscopy Experience*	93
The Man's Workup	99
Record of Semen Analyses	105
ESSAY: *I Gave at the Office*	108

SECTION III
YOUR INFERTILITY TREATMENT

Introduction to Section III	116
Do You Have a Diagnosis? Yes	117
Do You Have a Diagnosis? No	120
Your Infertility Treatment Is Planned	123
Reassessing Your Treatment	127
Infertility in Everyday Living	129
ESSAY: *Surely THIS Will be the Month*	132
ESSAY: *Want to Know a Secret?*	140
ESSAY: *I Often Ask Myself*	145
ESSAY: *If He'd Just Let Me Get Pregnant*	145
Taking a Break	146
Support Groups	148
When Counseling Could Help	149
Commonly Prescribed Treatments: What to Expect	151

Essay: *Be Aware, Don't Be Scared*	153
Essay: *I Just Needed a Little Help*	157
DES Exposure	168
Essay: *DES-Related Infertility*	170
A Warning: Pelvic Inflammatory Disease	171
The Special Problem of Miscarriage	171
Essay: *Miscarriage*	176
Commonly Prescribed Treatments For Men: What to Expect	177
Treatment for Both Partners	182
Essay: *With a Full Bladder and Your Heart in Your Throat*	193
Pregnancy After Infertility	194
Essay: *Does This Mean My Infertility is Resolved?*	196
Essay: *I Was Looking at a Stranger*	197

Section IV
The Alternatives

Introduction to Section IV	200
Look Ahead to Choices	201
Talking About Your Alternatives	201
The Need to Grieve	203
Poem: *Imaginary Child*	206
Considering Alternatives: The Best Interests of . . . Whom?	206
Artificial Insemination, Donor (AID)	207
Essay: *I Must Tell Someone*	214
Surrogate Parenting	215
Alternatives to the Alternatives: Of Eggs and Embryos	218
Deciding to End Medical Treatment	221
Essay: *The Relief From the Burden Was Palpable*	223
Adoption	225
Essay: *Are You Ready to be a Mom?*	233
Childfree Living	235
Essay: *Instead We Have Found Each Other*	242
Essay: *The Happiest Place on Earth*	244
Appendix	246
Reading Up on Infertility	246
Insurance and Cost Recovery	249

Insurance Policy Information at a Glance	253
Record of Insurance Claims	255
Record of Basal Body Temperature	256
Resources: Important Names and Addresses	258
Doctors, Hospitals, and Clinics	258
Laboratories	259
Medication Records	259
Bibliography	264
Index	267

Acknowledgments

I want to thank the dedicated men and women who have contributed essays to this book. Corresponding with these wonderful people has enriched my life. I'm deeply indebted to each of them. They were many days when a letter from one of them provided me with the strength I needed to keep working on this sometimes difficult project. Their patience, their warmth, their friendship, and their genuine concern for others restored my faith more than once. Their support made this book possible.

I thank my agent Vicky Bijur, of Charlotte Sheedy Literary Agency, for her amazing tenacity. Both Vicky and Charlotte recognized the worth of this project from its inception, and both were always positive that it would be published, even when I was not.

My editor, Stacy Prince, has stood by me with trust and good humor. Her enthusiasm for this book recharged my batteries each time I spoke to her. Her guidance enabled me to clarify my ideas and helped me to articulate the reasons why I wanted to write this book. Her faith in me, and her friendship, are very special.

Linda Pittman's experience as a nurse-practitioner in a busy infertility practice made her an ideal consultant to read my manuscript. But it is her ebullience, her clear vision, and her down-to-earth common sense about infertility that I value even more. Her great concern for her patients' well-being came through in every piece of advice she has given me. For these qualities, I thank her.

My beloved husband, Brian Rose, has weathered quite a remarkable storm along with me—both our experience with infertility and my compulsion to write about it! He encouraged me to pursue this project because he recognized immediately how much I needed to do so. And though there were many months when I was sure this book would never happen, Brian always helped me to persevere.

I also want to give special thanks to my wonderful sister, Elizabeth Frenchman, whose love and support never fails to amaze me. Merci, ma soeur.

Oh, and thank you, Sniffy, for keeping me company through the lonely hours of writing and for eating about half my research materials.

Brooklyn, New York
March 1988

Foreword

Infertile couples seeking to solve their problem are indeed confronted with an enormous, bewildering maze. You can't just go to the family doctor expecting him or her to have any significant knowledge of the highly specialized care you need. Nor can you necessarily trust his or her recommendation of which infertility specialist to see.

Even if you are lucky enough to locate a good doctor or clinic, you are certain to become confused by the complexity of tasks you have to perform in a coordinated and synchronized fashion as part of your treatment. Infertility is not a problem that can be managed by getting a few blood tests, a few x-rays, and then going on some medication. Whenever I have to break the reality of treatment schedules to the uninitiated infertility patient and see the disbelief in her eyes, I feel as if some teacher is in the room writing a lesson plan on a blackboard with a squeaky piece of chalk.

With just a simple cycle of stimulating ovulation, for example, a woman will have to make daily trips to the hospital early in the morning. She'll have to have her blood drawn for estrogen and LH levels, undergo an ultrasound examination to evaluate the quality and size of her egg follicles, and have a cervical mucus exam. Then she'll come back in the afternoon for a shot, the dosage of which was determined by the results of the morning's tests. This can go on for eight to twelve days in any cycle. Then, when her eggs are ripe, she has to have another shot, this one triggering ovulation. Her doctor might tell her to have intercourse with her husband (after abstaining for the previous week, of course), or he might ask her to bring her husband in at a precisely scheduled time so he can masturbate into a jar and have his sperm "washed" so they can be injected, through a catheter, directly into her uterus. This is one of the "simple" options, short of the more advanced, "high tech" treatments that might provide her better chances of success.

It is no wonder that many couples seem almost relieved if they are told that, rather than have to go through all this, they will simply need some surgery to correct their infertility problems. Surgery is painful and scary, but at least (so a couple may think) you go into the hospital, get it done, and then you can get pregnant.

Unfortunately, that's not the way it works. Even if the problem is one that requires surgery, the operation (or operations) is usually only the beginning. In fact, sometimes surgery is really inadvisable, but the patient doesn't know that the operation will not only get her no closer to her goal of getting pregnant, but may actually hurt her chances.

Furthermore, this medical side of infertility is only one aspect of the experience. The emotional and financial burdens on an infertile couple striving to become pregnant can be quite intense. It is easy to feel depressed, unfairly victimized, and alone when you see friends all around you getting pregnant almost effortlessly, while you as a couple are torn apart from the sheer exhaustion of trying to figure your way out of this maze. But the fact of the matter is that *you are not alone.* Twenty-five percent of couples in their thirties are infertile.

Ironically, only one percent of teenagers suffer this problem. This means that from your teen years through your twenties and thirties, there is a twenty-five-fold increase in your chance of having an infertility problem. It seems cruel that nature makes us most fertile at the age when we can least handle a baby and we are desperately trying *not* to get pregnant—yet after our careers are established, we are comfortable with our lives, and we have made the mature decision to start a family, the odds are one in four that we won't be able to do it. Not, at least, without medical help of some kind. It's crazy, but if you have taken a responsible attitude about your future, it seems you are punished by the increased chances of infertility. Even worse is the fact that you are likely to hear insensitive wise-cracks suggesting that somehow you are to blame yourself for "waiting so long." But you don't know that you wouldn't have faced the same problems if you'd been ready to get pregnant ten years ago, and you certainly did not walk into this maze on purpose.

Fortunately, there is a way out of the maze, and it is outlined in this book. It is written by someone who has been there, who has experienced the same anxiety that you are experiencing. *The Infertility Maze* will walk you through the entire experience of infertility, from finding a specialist to resolution, making you aware of the various alternatives available to you. If you have a clear picture of the entire process, you'll be more likely to make the best choices.

My experience has been that the patients who become knowledgeable and participate with me in their treatments are the ones most likely to get pregnant. So read as much as you can about infertility, and about the many and sometimes complex treatments now available to you. The better educated you become, the more you will be able to work with your doctor to develop an effective treatment plan. It helps to already be familiar with some of the options he or she suggests and to be able to ask intelligent questions. And even if you don't get pregnant, you will at least feel satisfied that you fully understand your condition and did your best, and that knowledge will be your strength.

Sherman J. Silber, M.D.
St. Luke's Hospital
St. Louis, Missouri

Introduction

What Is the Infertility Maze?

When you're caught in a maze you have no way of keeping your position in perspective—you can't see what's ahead of you. You may feel trapped and helpless. You could wander the same paths again and again, unable to prevent it. You consider yourself isolated and alone with no one alongside you to show you the way. At times you wonder if you will ever find the right path out of the maze, and you may become discouraged.

Grappling with infertility is a lot like trying to find the way out of a complex maze. Which way to the best doctors? What tests are around this corner? Does that path lead to effective treatment? What options can be utilized so that the way out can be found at last?

This book was designed to give infertile couples a complete look at the infertility experience from beginning to resolution, and to help them negotiate their way through the maze as efficiently as possible. Frequently, when couples realize that they're having difficulty conceiving, they simply don't know what to do. They may rely on age-old home remedies, or allow their actions to be controlled by myths and misinformation. They may not know which doctors can help them, or how to find them, or what to ask them. They may endure time-consuming or inappropriate therapies. They may not be aware of alternative ways to build a family, or they may not understand what the alternatives are really like. As a result of these troubles, they may lose heart and they may lose hope. This doesn't have to happen.

In this book you will find a step-by-step guide to help you discover your best way out of the infertility maze. It covers all phases of the infertility experience, medical, emotional, and practical.

Infertility isn't just a run-of-the-mill medical condition with a simple solution. This is a problem that affects two people. It brings with it fear, anxiety, anger, guilt, embarrassment, grief—and in the end, hope. It's a problem that reaches deep into your emotional life and invades your intimate relationship. Infertility can steal away all your attention and your energy. It can also require a great deal of your time and money. It can demand unprecedented commitment. It may become your obsession.

Resolving infertility is a process that must be worked through. You can't just push a button and make everything all right again, much as you would wish it.

When infertility is discovered, emotional changes can alter your view of the world, your relationship with your partner, even your attitude toward the baby you long for. It takes time and effort to recover from this setback, however temporary it may be. You must be willing to expend this effort, to take this time. If you do, you will resolve your infertility in a way that is right for you. *The Infertility Maze* will show you that infertility is a difficult condition, yes, but one you can learn about, cope with, and resolve.

Trying to encompass the total infertility experience between the covers of one book is a challenging task. There are so many aspects to infertility, ranging from financial worries to spiritual crises. And every aspect demands attention, often simultaneously.

This book contains advice and guidelines that touch upon the diverse problems infertility can cause. There are four main sections to the book, which correspond to stages commonly experienced in working through infertility. You may recognize your own situation in one of the following stages.

First, a couple realizes that becoming pregnant is taking more time than they had expected. This realization is often accompanied by anxiety and feelings of bewilderment. The first section will outline what can be done even at this early stage, answer the most common worries about infertility, and help you search for the proper medical care.

The second section helps you evaluate your chosen specialist and describes the common tests that are given to discover infertility in both men and women. The foundation of any medical care for infertility is good communication between doctor and patient. Feeling frightened or sad, infertility patients often need some help in knowing what to expect, what to plan for, and what to ask. The communication processes within the couple itself may also need some help during this stressful time. In this section you will find help in dealing with your disrupted lives.

Section three describes the many treatments commonly prescribed for infertility problems, and lets you know what you can expect from them. Again, you'll learn what to ask your doctor. If you have suffered miscarriages, or fear you may suffer one, you can read about this special problem in this section.

The last section describes the processes couples go through in discovering which alternatives can help them resolve their infertility. There are options that involve controversy, options that are traditional, and one option that acknowledges that some couples can happily live childfree.

At the back of the book you will find an appendix of important practical

INTRODUCTION

help. There is a list of books to read, addresses of resources that can send you more information, organizations you can join. There are extra basal body temperature charts, should you need them. There are pages for you to jot down names of doctors, labs, hospitals. There is a simple system for keeping track of your insurance reimbursements.

The Infertility Maze is a book that recognizes that infertility affects the spirit as well as the body. The discovery of infertility is often accompanied by a feeling of isolation and loneliness as couples begin to feel cut off from the fertile world. To help alleviate this feeling, included throughout this book are essays written by men and women who have experienced infertility and want to share their thoughts. These personal stories and bits of advice can help you to feel a sense of fellowship and to realize that you're not alone in this struggle.

Plus, there are cartoons scattered throughout the book that anyone going through infertility can identify with. The sadness of infertility is often tempered by amazing absurdities, and these cartoons bring out the bittersweet side of this experience.

The most important theme running through this book is that you should try to understand and follow your doctor's thinking as you are both tested and treated for infertility. Being a well-informed and curious patient brings many benefits. First, if you learn about your condition and discuss it actively with your doctor, you help to dispel your apprehensions based on fears of the unknown. To know about the tests and treatments you face helps this whole process to seem less frightening. You will be able to ask your questions more specifically, and you'll be better able to understand the answers you receive. You will keep your doctor on her toes! Ask any infertility specialist and you'll hear how actively most infertility patients involve themselves in their cases.

Following along with your tests and treatments is important for another reason. Infertility is not a life-threatening condition in most instances. You may have never discovered your problem had you not begun trying to become pregnant. The way you are tested and treated for infertility is therefore pretty much elective—that is, it is up to you to give the go-ahead for how your case is handled. In addition, the doctor needs essential information from you so that tests and treatments can be scheduled properly. You are a vital member of your own medical team! The more you understand, the more you can participate in the decision making that directly affects your life.

You should have a good grasp of your situation for another reason. You will want to be able to recognize when it's time to try a different treatment or even to change doctors. These major decisions are up to you alone, and seeing their necessity is vitally important if you feel your case is going nowhere. Passive trust in your doctor has no place in infertility treatment.

Infertility can bring a feeling of frustration and helplessness. This comes from the loss of control of your life choices that you are experiencing. Your decision to become a parent has been deferred. You are constantly under a doctor's care, which even extends to regulation of your sex life. While there's little you can do to directly change these stresses, you can regain some sense of control by learning as much as you can about what's happening to you. You will not feel manipulated by the medical community because you will understand the thinking behind your treatment. Your decisions will be based on facts, not fears. Plus, participating in this way will give you something concrete to do during a time when you're probably feeling impatient and nervous. Reading, talking, asking, learning, deciding—all these activities are better than sitting on your hands, going crazy!

This book will show you how you can begin to take an active role in resolving your infertility. You can find out what questions to ask the doctor, how to find reading material, how to hold constructive discussions together. Doing all this will not miraculously "cure" you, but it will help you feel better in the meantime. And feeling better along the way is just as important as finding the right resolution.

Every infertility experience is different. For that reason, I have purposely omitted any discussion of the success rates of various procedures; not only are the statistics subject to change, but only your doctor can give you a reasonable assessment of how each procedure will work for you. (I have also left out information on how much each of the procedures will cost you, as it can vary widely depending on where you live and how much is covered by your insurance company.) Each case progresses at its own pace, as set by the physical and emotional capabilities and limitations of the couple. Although there is no timetable you can follow absolutely, you can make some efforts to help resolve your infertility and find your way out of the maze at last.

Improve communication between you and your doctor. Keep up with your workup test results and follow your doctor's train of thought as treatment is planned. Read about reproduction, fertility, and infertility, and improve your understanding of your own case. Ask vital questions, and ask the small questions, too. Help your doctor help you by asking questions whenever you have a problem. Set a loose timetable for treatment expectations, and ask about alternative treatments should they be needed. Let your doctor know your specific needs and how you are doing emotionally as well as physically. Attend important medical appointments with your partner whenever possible.

Make sure both partners are thoroughly checked for the major causes of infertility. It is important to avoid a hit-or-miss investigation of your infertility problem. In approximately 20 percent of cases, both partners contribute to a couple's infertility, so both of you must be examined. In addition, finding one infertility problem, especially a minor one, does not automatically eliminate the possibility that others may also be present. You may lose valuable time if your workups are halted when one problem is found in one partner. This incomplete examination could come back to haunt you should further problems crop up later, after you think you are "cured." Knowing that you both have been thoroughly examined should help your peace of mind, too.

Strive for frank and nonjudgmental communication between partners. Making the difficult decisions connected with infertility will be a little easier if you agree to listen to each other as well as talk to each other. Finding the answers that are right for you can only happen if you both are honest and open about your personal feelings. Disagreements will happen and it may sometimes take hard work to overcome them. In improving your communication skills together you not only help yourselves find your way out of the infertility maze, but you strengthen your relationship for the future.

Gain perspective on the infertility experience as a whole. Working through an infertility problem is a process with a beginning and a resolution. It takes some couples months to progress emotionally through infertility, but often it can take longer. Your individual needs will determine the pace of your resolution. Don't rush yourself into a decision that may not be right for you. And don't hesitate to ask for help if you are afraid that you've gotten stuck. Looking at the infertility experience as a whole will help you to figure out what steps you may need to take in order to keep progressing toward resolution. You will make it!

Support and respect one another. While you are trying for a child, don't neglect your relationship. It is just as important to preserve a good quality of life for yourselves now, even as you concentrate on building your future. This can be done by keeping honesty, warmth, and respect as daily goals to strive for as you interact. This means fighting as fairly as you can, giving empathy and sympathy to each other, eliminating recriminations, and not being threatened by sincere disagreements. Infertility has struck you as a couple, but you remain individuals. Your reactions will differ sometimes and you must cope with these differences as you search for your resolution.

Reach out to RESOLVE. Finding the organization RESOLVE early in your infertility experience is one of the best things you can do for yourselves. RESOLVE, Inc., is a nonprofit organization dedicated to helping people learn about and overcome infertility. A membership offers you invaluable information, newsletters, support groups, contact persons, and referrals to skilled and appropriate medical care. The members of RESOLVE are caring, warm people who want to help one another. You can receive this help in whatever form you are able to accept it, including: receiving information and newsletters through the mail, calling a telephone contact person to ask a question, attending scheduled meetings or support groups in your area. Just knowing that there is an organization to help couples cope with infertility can be a relief in itself! This book will continuously recommend the help that RESOLVE members can receive, simply because it can be a lifesaver.

There will be days when you wonder if you will ever live through all of this, if your relationship will survive, if you'll ever find resolution. I hope this book will lend you the advice and perspective you need to realize that yes, indeed, you will.

SECTION I
When You Realize You Have a Problem

*t*his first section is designed to help you if you're just beginning to worry about your ability to have a baby.

Some couples are caught offguard by this realization, while others have long suspected or feared that they might have trouble. But regardless of how you arrived at this realization, the worries are the same—are we too old, should we just relax, who do we call, what can we do now?

In this section you will find the most common worries couples have about infertility and read the facts about those worries. Knowing these facts will help you to either stop worrying or decide to see a doctor. Either action is much more positive than continuing to be anxious.

You'll read advice on how to find a good doctor, how to set up your initial appointment with a specialist, and the things you can do to prepare for it. Plus, this section shows you how to begin tracking ovulation yourselves, at home, to find the best days for conception.

Section I also covers some of the most common advice you'll hear from friends and relatives who mean well, but are misinformed. The familiar "Relax!" is actually not helpful at all. Nor is the time-honored advice to first adopt a child. You'll read here why this is so.

Remember, even if it is taking you a while to become pregnant, there may not be anything wrong. You may just need more time to conceive. In this section you can read about how to come to a better understanding of this whole process, so that you can judge for yourselves what you should do about getting pregnant—and when to do it.

Are You Worried That You Might Not Be Able to Have a Baby?

As you make your happy plans, you take for granted that you'll get pregnant before long, right? Nobody thinks infertility could happen to them—it's something that hits other people. Yet in the back of your mind, you begin wondering about some of the things you've been reading, and worrying about what you've heard about having babies these days.

And these days, it may take only a few months of trying before we start worrying. Since we hear so much about the "biological clock" (oh, that phrase!) or toxic contamination, stress, or strange diseases, it's no surprise that we become concerned so soon.

Simply being admonished not to worry won't stop your questions. You need answers to the specific problems you are concerned about, logic to explain away the confusion, courage to face your fears. "Stop it, you're just being silly!" repeated to yourself dozens of times a day won't do it. Being told to relax and take a trip doesn't help either.

Anxiety about infertility doesn't go away by magic. It must be confronted, analyzed, and explained, and only then does it recede. Even on a subject as painful and scary as infertility, the unknown details of the subject are usually more frightening than facing the reality.

The Questions You Worry About

Here are some of the major reasons why people worry about infertility, and something you can learn or do about each:

Are you worried because of your age?

Knowing something about the relationship of age to fertility will help here. It is true that:

- peak fertility is generally acknowledged to be between the ages of twenty and twenty-five, for both men and women.
- after age twenty-five, a woman's ability to readily conceive begins to slightly taper off.
- after age thirty, a woman's fertility begins to drop more rapidly, and the risk of complications begins to go up.

Generally, you should realize that natural conception takes time, and the amount of time varies with the individuals. If you are in your early to mid-twenties, the average amount of time is around six months. If you are in your early to mid-thirties it could be up to or past a year. Keep in mind, though, that the problem with these generalizations is that there are ALWAYS lots of exceptions. There could be nothing wrong with a twenty-five-year-old who needs a full year to conceive, just as a thirty-eight-year-old may only need two months.

Natural conception needs time to work. This sounds like glib advice, but there are rules of thumb you can think about:

- **Try to balance** your age with the amount of time you've been trying. Then think about your level of personal concern. Listen to your inner voice, and if you are still worried after noting these age generalities, then it's time to talk to a doctor.

- **If you are** over thirty, or your spouse is over thirty, you should feel no hesitation if you'd like to consult a doctor. Don't let a doctor hush you up and send you away, even if you've been trying for only six months. You can at least get started on a gradual workup. If your doctor is reluctant to treat you, you should go to another doctor.

- **You have the** right to have your concerns taken seriously, no matter what your age.

Are you worried because you've already been trying for a while and nothing's happening?

The definition of infertility used in America is the inability to conceive and carry to term a pregnancy after one full year of unprotected intercourse.

This definition was articulated in the days when most women began childbearing in the most fertile years of their twenties, before so many women delayed this effort in order to start careers or live other kinds of lives. Still, if you are in your mid-twenties, this definition probably does fit you. You won't be "official" until at least a year has passed, and some doctors may not see you as a serious infertility patient for that reason.

If you aren't in the optimum fertility age bracket, does that definition apply? Probably not, but there's no definition in use for older women, so you will have to decide for yourself when you should become concerned and when to see a doctor.

"Trying for a while" is a vague term, and each couple will have an inner sense of how much time they feel comfortable with. For a couple in their mid-thirties, "a while" could mean six months. But for a younger couple, or any couple feeling optimistic, the realization that they've been trying for a while may not come for well over a year. For couples trying on a very casual basis, this could even be five years.

In his book *How to Get Pregnant*, Dr. Sherman Silber provides a clear discussion of how long it might take a couple to conceive. Dr. Silber reports that any fertile woman has 20 percent odds of conceiving during any given month. Therefore, you must give yourselves a decent amount of time for this flip of the coin to catch up with you.

It isn't easy to just sit by and wait for nature to take its course, especially when there's so much technology to help us out. But realize that you could save yourself a lot of time, worry, and money if you can wait and see a bit longer.

Again, balance your age and time you've been trying against that inner voice that might tell you to worry. Are you still concerned, even against all this common sense? You still have the right to have all your questions answered by a doctor. And you have a right to say when.

Are you worried because of the scary things you've been reading about the high incidence of infertility?

This problem is certainly getting more publicity these days. Is it media hype, or is there truth to these stories? How common is infertility?

Statistics on the incidence of infertility range from a low estimate of 8.5 percent to the generally accepted figure of 15 percent to a high of almost 20 percent. Most health-care professionals agree that about one-sixth of couples trying to have a baby have trouble doing so.

Because baby boomers are such a big bulge in the general population, anything they do, they do in big numbers. So, if one-sixth of them are defined as infertile, it begins to make news. What's more, knowledge of what causes infertility problems is increasing all the time and this, too, makes news. We know more about reproductive processes, diseases, environmental factors, occupational hazards, and even man-made problems that interfere with fertility. Infertility is greatly publicized because of the various scientific, legal, and ethical questions brought out by the newest technological solutions. All these reports may make infertility seem even more common than it actually is.

It's true, infertility is common. But that doesn't mean you are going to "catch" it. Read about the causes of infertility, and you will begin to see if any factors may apply to you. You may want to ask your doctor a few quick questions just to ease your mind—and that's fine.

Are you worried because you've had trouble with your periods in the past?

To most of us, this would be the most obvious sign there might be a problem.

If you now have very irregular or very crampy periods, or you do not menstruate at all, then yes, you should see a doctor right away. You might feel comfortable just going over this with your regular gynecologist, who ought to know your history anyway. In light of your desire for pregnancy, this problem needs urgent attention.

Sometimes the solution to this problem is simple and your gynecologist will be well able to handle it. If it looks to your doctor like your problem is more complex, you can be referred to the proper specialist or begin to look for one yourself. Don't be shy about asking exactly what the problem is and what can be done about it.

If you are not having periods at all, this is a serious problem. Could it be caused by extreme amounts of exercise, dieting, or great stress? Talk over these possibilities with your doctor.

If your problem periods are in your distant past, you may not have much to worry about. Irregular periods are normal in young girls in the first year or so of menstruation. But do think back over the years and see if your periods have changed significantly in character (length, amount of flow, cramps, clotting) since they settled down. Talk over any changes you recall with the doctor.

Are you worried because you've been diagnosed in the past with a condition or disease that you now realize can be a factor in fertility?

This is another good reason to talk to your doctor right away if you're trying to become pregnant. Again, having a regular relationship with a gynecologist will help, because your history will already be known. If you don't have a regular gyn, start going to one, and bring her up to date pronto.

For women, these factors ought to be seriously considered if any apply to you: endometriosis, pelvic infections or pelvic inflammatory disease, sexually transmitted diseases, complications from birth control use (irregular periods following use of the Pill, use of an IUD), and multiple abortions (more than two, or one from which you may not have healed properly). Consider also: did your mother take the drug DES while she was pregnant with you? Have you had abdominal surgery? Have you taken any medications for a protracted period of time?

For men, factors to think about include: mumps after puberty, surgery in the lower abdomen, sexually transmitted diseases, swelling in the groin, undescended testicle, and protracted use of medications.

THESE FACTORS DO NOT MEAN THAT YOU ARE NOW INFERTILE. But they can give your doctors a warning flag to search further if you are having a problem conceiving.

Be sure your doctor is listening to you carefully and fully questioning you regarding your medical history. If you are told that these factors have been well considered and have not impaired your fertility, you can ask for complete explanations to settle your mind. If you're still worried, ask what tests could apply to your situation. It's a big step to ask for a test yourself, but if you must know you're OK, sometimes this is the only way.

Are you worried because of you or your partner's sexual history, your past or present lifestyle, or because of occupational hazards?

- **If you are** worried about the legacy of many past sexual encounters, try to distinguish if this is just guilt talking or if you have a need for concern. The only real worry you might have in this situation is the possibility that you or your partner may have contracted a sexually transmitted disease (STD), perhaps more than once. It's possible to have an STD and not even realize it. For example, the disease chlamydia is now recognized as very widespread, often symptomless, and a real cause of damage to fertility. If you think you may now have an STD, see the doctor without delay.

- **Did you use** the Pill or an IUD before trying to become pregnant? If these birth control devices did not cause any complications, there should be no reason for you to worry. Was your IUD removed with no problem? Did your periods resume normally after you discontinued the Pill? Talk to your doctor if you're wondering about them.

- **Do you smoke,** drink, use "recreational" drugs? A little? A lot? Then, but not now?

Because we read about how bad smoking and drinking are for the already pregnant woman, it's easy to worry that these habits also inhibit fertility. Smoking is beginning to emerge as a factor in infertility, although no major studies confirm this. (You shouldn't be smoking in any event.) Keeping drinking to a very modest level is always smart, too.

In men, smoking hasn't officially been connected to impaired fertility, but why do it? Excessive drinking is thought to be a factor in reduced sperm quality, and too much drink can cause impotence, so if alcohol is an important daily habit with you, talk about it with your doctor.

Smoking marijuana has also been connected with a reduced quality of sperm in heavy or regular users. If either of you is using drugs heavily or regularly, there is more being impaired in your life than just your fertility. You must be frank with your doctor about your use of drugs of any type. And don't just talk about how drug use is affecting your bodies; try to discover your motives, and get hold of your habit now.

- **Isn't this polluted** world a cause of infertility? What about occupational hazards?

We keep reading vague references to "environmental factors," but what are they? It's a tough question to answer because of contradictory studies, defensive protests from industrial polluters, and the small amount of time we've had to even study this problem. Some things we do know. If you or your partner is regularly exposed to toxic chemicals or radiation on the job, be concerned. If you live in a very heavily industrialized region, you might look into what pollutants may be in your air and water. You probably have little cause for concern, but if you want to quit worrying, consult a fertility specialist and ask up front about environment and fertility. Many specialists believe environmental factors contribute to reduced sperm counts or quality in men and possibly to miscarriages in women. A simple semen analysis could put your mind at rest.

In men, exposure to heat on the job could interfere with good sperm production. Sitting all day or working in front of a blast furnace could have the same effect. Change jobs? That sounds extreme, but sometimes just changing to looser boxer undershorts can help. Talk about your job routine with the doctor.

Are you worried because you don't really understand fully how your bodies work to produce a baby, and you're too embarrassed to ask?

It's amazing how complicated reproduction is once you stop to look at it. Most of us get through high school health class, then proceed to forget about our

WHEN YOU REALIZE YOU HAVE A PROBLEM

reproductive systems. We use birth control, sure, but when it comes time to reverse gears and try for a baby, do we know what's going on? Even if you've got a Ph.D., you may not be aware of all the physiological and hormonal factors involved in successful conception, pregnancy, and birth:

- a healthy egg produced by the woman and picked up by the end of the fallopian tube
- healthy, active sperm in sufficient numbers
- sperm deposited in the right spot, at the right time of the woman's cycle
- open (patent) fallopian tubes
- ability of sperm to swim in good cervical mucus through the cervix to fallopian tubes, penetrate egg, fertilize it
- ability of fertilized egg to travel down tube, into uterus, and implant
- a strong, flexible uterus and healthy, normally formed cervix
- correct hormone levels to support pregnancy
- time to get all these factors into sync for a successful pregnancy

Read about the male and female reproductive systems. Going over these physiological facts will help you visualize what you're doing, and assist you in discussing your questions with the doctor.

Are you worried that you "might not be doing it right"?

In trying to get pregnant, there isn't one right way to make love with your partner in order to conceive. When all factors are normal for fertility, you can become pregnant by making love in all kinds of positions, in any room of the house, no matter what record is on the stereo. If you learn more about how your bodies work together, you'll stop worrying about what you're doing and if it's "right."

However, if you want to enhance your chances every bit that you can, you should certainly learn to recognize what days of the month are your fertile ones and plan to make love around that time. Plus, some doctors advise that the old-fashioned missionary position seems to direct the most sperm to the optimum place in the vagina. But if you find this recommendation too stressful, remember that it's not necessary Having the woman remain lying down for fifteen to thirty mmutes afterward can help the sperm swim along, too. You don't *have* to stand on your head. Read ahead to how to recognize fertile days.

Are you worried because people you know are starting their families, and their pregnancies and children make you feel different? Are relatives or friends starting to needle you?

It's very hard to shake off the societal pressure to reproduce, that peer pressure to join the club when others around you are already pregnant. Fending off requests for grandchildren can be particularly difficult when you are just starting to try and aren't successful right away. If feeling pressure from others is starting to make you worry about infertility, examine your feelings carefully. Is this outside interference the only cause of your worries about conception? If it is, you must take a deep breath and give nature some more time. Can you tell your friends to knock off the teasing? Are you comfortable saying, "We're working on it"? Or, try telling your family to relax before they have a chance to tell you!

If this outside pressure echoes your own growing worries about how long this ought to take, call your doctor and discuss your questions directly. Go over the reasons for fertility problems previously listed, and see if there might be any real basis for the delay—or if you're just impatient.

Are you worried because you feel so desperate for a baby already?

Infertility is a problem of life-crisis stature. It is natural to feel upset, anxious, or unhappy. Don't panic because you're feeling sad or out of sorts about it. If your worry about conception is bordering on desperation, you need reassurance that you're OK. Talk to your doctor right away and assess your need for a fertility workup. Knowing you are doing something concrete about it can make you feel more in control of your life. Consult with your gynecologist or begin investigating names of fertility specialists. It often takes many weeks, even months, to get a first appointment with a specialist, but at least you can lay the groundwork for a possible future appointment now—just in case.

Making an appointment with the doctor doesn't mean you're infertile. It means you are doing the safe, smart thing to insure that possible problems can be detected early, and that will help you to worry less.

This done, think again about why you are feeling so desperate. If you have indeed been trying for quite some time, it is very understandable. But if you're just getting started and you're still very jittery, try looking more closely at why this may be so:

- **achievement anxiety**—Our work ethic teaches us that if we do the right things and work hard, we will invariably achieve success. Unfortunately, nature doesn't necessarily operate on the same principles as we do. Do you overachieve in other parts of your life? Could this be carrying over to your quest for pregnancy?
- **impatience**—This is a high-speed world. Everything seems to be instantaneous. You must try to cool it and wait out a decent period of time for your attempts at pregnancy to have a chance at success. See the earlier discussion of the odds in the subsection, "Trying for a while."
- **acquisitiveness**—Don't turn your hoped-for baby into a commodity. Let the advertisers and merchandisers do that. Give your baby a sweet, human face in your imagination, and give her or him the chance to come to you in its own time.

Realize that you may be attaching a great symbolic importance to this effort to conceive or to the baby itself. Everybody does. But this "hidden agenda" might be the cause of your intense anxiety. If your worries are getting the better of you, you have the right to go to your doctor and ask all your questions. But you may be worried about more than making babies: saving your marriage, growing up, the decision to have a child in the first place. Recognition of these possible reasons will help you become more objective and may calm you down, too.

Are you worried because you feel all alone and don't have anybody to talk to about infertility, or to answer all the "stupid" questions?

You are not alone. Someone you know also has this worry. It's just that infertility isn't a subject that most people feel comfortable talking about. Plus, we are often taught not to complain, to keep our anxieties to ourselves.

If you are worried that you might be infertile, having your friends, relatives, and even doctors brush it off at first is no help. But this sometimes happens. You have a right to have your questions addressed seriously, and sometimes it will be up to you to find your own answers. There is a way for you to find information, have questions answered, get referrals for doctors and specialists, even find counseling and support groups for infertility. A national organization called RESOLVE, Inc., was formed especially to address the problems of infertility.

RESOLVE has chapters all over the country. Even if your area doesn't have one, RESOLVE has a network of "contact persons" you can speak to. Even if you aren't ready to assume you have a fertility problem, nobody at RESOLVE will chide you if you just want to ask questions. To reach RESOLVE:

>RESOLVE, INC.
>5 Water Street
>Arlington, Massachusetts 02174
>(617) 643-2424

Ask how to contact the chapter nearest you, and consider supporting their efforts by sending a donation or joining yourself. Just knowing that there's a network of caring, dedicated professonals and volunteers ready to help you build your family can make all the difference in the world. You are not alone!

A Future Without Children

DOROTHY J. HAGERTY

I'm not really sure when we felt the realization that we were an infertile couple. I did not have my first menstrual period until I was sixteen, and then it was very sporadic. Five years after my husband and I were married, we felt that we were ready to start a family. After being off the Pill for a year without a conception, I consulted my gynecologist. My endometrial biopsy was normal and the hysterosalpingogram indicated that I might have a blocked tube. While I went through this testing, my husband had a semen analysis done. The results showed he had a very low count with virtually no motility. At that point all of my testing was stopped, and we concentrated on correcting my husband's condition. After two years of tests and medications (Clomid) for him, the results were not much better than his first count.

I believe it was at this point that we first realized that not everything could be corrected or treated with medication, and we could be looking at a future without children. We reacted with all the typical emotions of anger, disbelief, confusion, mistrust, hurt, pity, and fear. We were angry at our relatives and friends who had no trouble having children, and we grew very impatient with the thousands of questions from those close to us. How could this be happening to us? My husband was the most disappointed and felt our childlessness was his fault. I feel it is very important to stress that infertility is not an individual problem—it is a couple's problem. Neither of you is to be blamed solely. If you allow this bitterness to grow inside of you, it could hurt you and possibly hurt your marriage.

My husband's specialist informed us of four possible options considering my husband's condition. One of the possiblities was that by chance he might get me pregnant; if that didn't work, we would need to consider artificial insemination, in vitro fertilization, or adoption. We took several months to digest this blow and then I made an appointment with my infertility specialist to discuss my history and our medical options. Before my husband and I could make any decisions, we had to know where we stood. My specialist performed a laparoscopy and determined that I had no anatomical problems. However, I was not ovulating, and therefore needed drug therapy (Clomid) in order to conceive.

At this point, my husband and I needed to decide which direction we would take. After considerable thought we felt we had to go on trying. We couldn't give up that easily even if our options weren't ideal. At least we did have options. I started taking medication, and when my ovulatory cycle was regulated, we selected artificial insemination. That was one and a half years ago. The road has been a long one with many hills and valleys, but it's one we have not regretted traveling. There will never be guarantees for an infertile couple, and that can be very discouraging. If we can find solace and peace with our treatment for infertility, it is the fact that we did try and didn't give up. We will not have to look back and say, "What if . . . ?"

Does Worrying Affect Fertility? Should You Just "Relax"?

Don't feel bad if you're worried about infertility. It's natural to be concerned about the process of conception if you think you might have a problem.

Contrary to conventional wisdom, worry does not cause infertility. It's the infertility that causes the worry.

Over 90 percent of fertility problems can now be traced to a physical cause. The percentage has risen over the years, and as the physical causes are found, the old "relax" cure is steadily being replaced with treatments based in medical science. Is it then logical to expect that the 10 percent that remains unknown will be caused by those stress-related factors? Of course not. While there is probably some connection between the function of the hypothalamus (in the brain) and stress, there's just no proof that simple "relaxation" is all it takes to become pregnant. Science just hasn't finished its job yet. If you further apply logic, you'd see that there are lots of stressed-out women in this world who have no trouble getting pregnant.

Stress can tinker with your menstrual cycles, delay ovulation, and make intercourse difficult. But these are symptoms that you can see, something you can track. Your problem is not mysterious hocus-pocus, hidden away deep within your psyche.

If your anxiety over conception is messing up your cycles, being told to relax just isn't going to help. You must stop feeling guilty that you might be causing your own problem—because you aren't. Do everything you can do to help yourself, find competent and compassionate medical attention, and learn all you can. This won't help you relax and get pregnant, but it will help you feel better for your own sake. That's just as important.

Don't invent a cause-and-effect relationship that doesn't exist. Your worries aren't mysteriously making you infertile. Dealing with your worries as specifically as you can and finding out if there is any basis for them is the best thing you can do. If there is a basis, you can get help. If there really isn't, you can throw that nagging worry away at last. Resolve to eliminate as many of these anxieties as you can, one by one.

"Adopt, and You'll Get Pregnant."

Somebody we tell about our infertility worry will invariably know someone who:

- adopted, then got pregnant
- quit her job, then got pregnant
- started a new job, then got pregnant
- took a trip, then got pregnant
- gave up trying, then got pregnant

The inability to conceive readily is frightening to most people and is initially so mysterious, so unknowable. The ability to reproduce is taken for granted with such an intensity that we find the most logical parts of ourselves willing to believe in cause-and-effect relationships that just aren't there.

We all know the story of the explorer in the jungle who comes upon a village at the exact moment that the sun goes into eclipse. The villagers, frightened and unaware of natural laws, attribute the end of the eclipse and the restoration of sunlight to the visit of the explorer.

The villagers have given the explorer far more power than she really has, and the factor of coincidence is never considered. This story is analogous to "adopt and you'll get pregnant." As we search for an answer to our problem, we'll often hear from others how easy it is to get pregnant if we would only change jobs, move to a new house, etc.

What we and our friendly advisers are really doing is going for that nonexistent cause-and-effect relationship. We strongly wish that positive actions in other parts of our lives will bring the reward of pregnancy.

It's hard not to believe in the veracity of this advice: we all do know people who adopt, then get pregnant. So, what's going on? Is it coincidence or not? Will adoption make infertility go away? Did the explorer make the eclipse go away?

Studies show that there is an unexplained or "spontaneous" pregnancy occurrence in about 5 percent to 10 percent of all infertility cases. This means that the couple has gotten pregnant without intervention, for no apparent reason. In a study published by Leurgans and Lamb in 1979 in *The American Journal of Obstetrics and Gynecology,* the percentage of couples who become pregnant after adopting exactly matched the percentage who spontaneously conceived without adopting.

This phenomenon of spontaneous pregnancy is probably due to physical factors doctors haven't uncovered yet. Or, it could be that a couple is simply destined to take a certain amount of time to conceive. While they wait, they adopt or move or travel the world. Then when pregnancy occurs, it looks like the child, the new address, or the trip did it. It probably didn't.

It is true that beginning to occupy oneself with other matters and limiting one's obsession with fertility can diminish stress. The "relax, and . . ." factor comes in here again, but remember, stress is usually caused by infertility, not the reverse.

You can only gain by improving other parts of your life that infertility may have caused you to neglect. But enjoy your improved outlook on life, your new job, your new house for what it is—a step toward better living, not a bargaining tool for you to use against fate.

If we, the infertile, buy the argument that if we only would do the right thing, we would then conceive, what are we doing? Again, we're saying that we're causing our own infertility. This time, it's by the sin of omission. We are agreeing with the premise that by not doing just the right thing, we're causing or prolonging the problem. Oh, the guilt this can cause! This just adds to the stress of infertility and will make us feel worse instead of better.

Don't take on powers you don't really have. Keep in mind the medical facts and learn to distinguish them from these powerful myths. Tell your helpful friends and relatives the explorer/villagers story—if they're giving you this "cause-and-effect" explanation, they're behaving like those villagers did. The power you, the "explorer," will hold, then, is the power of knowledge and logic.

Do You Need a Specialist Yet?

If you think you have an infertility problem, should you go to a specialist right away? Can a good ob-gyn solve some of these problems at less expense? Does a general practitioner or internist know enough about reproduction to treat infertility, in men or women? Which doctors should be consulted for what?

There are many types of doctors you can turn to, and each will be described here. Read about what each can offer you.

Only you can decide how you want to have your problem investigated. First, what are your priorities? You may be looking for someone with the latest information and specific training in infertility treatment, in addition to someone with skill and experience. Plus, you want your investigation to be complete. You do not want to waste valuable time, especially if the woman is thirty or older. If these priorities describe your needs, consider looking for an infertility specialist right away. The search might take a few weeks of phone calls, questions, and waiting for a first appointment, but you will feel better knowing that you're going to the experts at the start.

However, some people don't feel quite ready to plunge in so quickly to a complete infertility investigation, or they feel they can't afford it yet. They may not even be sure that they have a problem. They may just need to talk things over with a trusted general practitioner or gynecologist before deciding to search further.

It won't hurt you to start out with a doctor less qualified than a specialist in infertility, and it may help to talk to a doctor who already knows your medical history. But bear in mind that should you need more expert advice, you will be referred to a specialist anyway.

As you go over your needs with your present doctor, be ready to ask about consulting a specialist, and see how open she is to your doing so. A doctor who is genuinely interested in your welfare will usually not object to this move. If you do start your infertility investigation with your current doctor, use the guidelines in this book to help you determine if and when you need to move on for more help.

Obstetrician-Gynecologist (Ob-Gyn)

Most people think first of the ob-gyn as the doctor to see when infertility is suspected. And in some cases, an ob-gyn could be all you need. Simple ovulation problems and infections, for example, are treated by these doctors every day. Plus, your doctor's familiarity with your history will serve as a good jumping-off point in the investigation.

If you choose to start with your ob-gyn, you should try to be as frank as you can. Ask, "Will you be able to test and treat my husband and me for infertility? Can you refer us to specialists if you cannot?" Your doctor's reaction to this question alone will give you information. A good ob-gyn will know when to send you on to a specialist and won't have any ego problems doing so.

Ob-Gyn—Infertility Specialist

The term "infertility specialist" is vague. Some gynecologists see only infertility patients and have gradually become specialists in this area of women's health care. Some are indeed very knowledgeable in this field and can treat patients expertly. But they have no official board certification hanging on the wall that states this. You must ask any specialist about her training and qualifications, but it's quite important with this kind of gynecologist. Unfortunately, there are overeager ob-gyns who may hang out the "infertility specialist" shingle but who do not have the expertise, so be careful.

Since this doctor may not have specific extra training in infertility, you must determine how "plugged in" to the field she really is. Ask about how this specialty evolved in the practice, and what practical experience and successes the doctor has had. This will help.

This type of doctor may also be an obstetrician. Ask. You might see pregnant women in the waiting room, which can be upsetting. But you may want your baby to be delivered by the doctor who helped you conceive it. Depending on how you feel about it, consider asking if separate hours are held for infertility and obstetrical patients.

This infertility specialist may be more likely to view the infertility as a problem of both partners until the reasons begin to be discovered. In a logical workup it's important for both partners to be involved for medical reasons as well as for your peace of mind.

Board-Certified Specialist in Reproductive Endocrinology/Infertility

This infertility specialist has completed a two-year fellowship in addition to the regular training necessary for gynecology. Endocrinology refers to hormones and the role they play in fertility, and that role is a big one. These infertility specialists are also qualified to perform microsurgery should the need arise.

These doctors are obviously the best formally trained specialists in infertility investigation. They may charge you more for the same services you'd get from a noncertified infertility specialist. However, being on the cutting edge of the field could be just what your case needs.

A specialist in reproductive endocrinology/infertility will investigate the woman very thoroughly, but might focus on the woman alone. Be sure the man's role is investigated too.

Involvement in research is a hallmark of many of these specialists. You might feel that your doctor is sometimes more involved with you as a case study than as a person. But knowing you're getting the benefit of the latest research can offset this problem for some patients. If you start to feel you're on an assembly line, try to speak up. Unfortunately, when consulting specialists, it's often up to the patient to demand more humane care.

Urologist

This specialist could be called the "man's doctor," and is largely the counterpart to the gynecologist. This physician treats the male reproductive and urinary tracts, and can give many of the tests and treatments needed for male infertility problems. A urologist may also be a surgeon.

Since these doctors treat only the man, they might be lopsided in their view of your infertility case. The woman should attend as many appointments as she can, and the doctor should always discuss your situation as a couple. Keep the urologist well-informed on the woman's workup and be sure the woman's physician knows all about what the urologist is doing.

Andrologist

This relatively new specialty is actually a subspecialty of urology. If it becomes apparent that there is a complex problem in the man that requires more intensive testing or drug therapy, you may be referred to an andrologist.

As with a urologist, the specialty here has a narrow focus, so it's up to the patients to insure that their total care is well-rounded and that all the doctors involved are talking to one another.

Infertility Clinics

You probably have heard about infertility clinics or fertility centers as the most advanced place to have a complete workup. These facilities get lots of publicity as breakthroughs in fertility technology (such as in vitro fertilization) are made. This publicity has a very strong appeal and this alone can get you to pick up the phone.

The experience of treatment in a clinic atmosphere varies, of course, but it is often different from treatment given by a private physician. You may not be seen by the same doctor all the time, as the specialists apply a "team" approach to your case. You might feel more anonymous as a result.

Regulation of clinics is vague in many states, so you should approach them with lots of questions. Find out the routine for a typical workup, costs, how many different doctors you might see. As they describe their services and success rates, ask for a thorough explanation. Ask if the clinic is involved in research and, if so, of what type.

In general, unless there is no private infertility specialist available who meets your needs, don't go first to the large clinics. They could be more involved with the advanced technologies of pregnancy induction, which you may not need. Try to go to a specialist in private practice, and if it is determined that you do need the services of such a clinic, you can be appropriately referred.

Many successful infertility specialists have long waiting lists for first-time appointments, but your doctor should see you promptly when you need attention thereafter. If you think you should start off with a specialist, then begin your search for one right away. If you find a specialist you'd like to see, make an appointment, even if it's for two months in advance. Find out the cancellation policy as you schedule it. If you change your mind later, or become pregnant, you can always cancel (be courteous and do it in plenty of time). As you continue to try to get pregnant, you can thus feel reassured that you aren't wasting any more precious time.

How to Find and Choose a Specialist

When you feel it's time to put yourselves in an expert's hands, choosing that expert looms as a tremendous task. Physicians hold a place of high respect in our society, and it's hard not to attribute great powers to them as we turn to them for help. This is an impulse you should try to resist as you evaluate several prospective doctors to help you find your infertility problem.

As you search for the right specialist, think of yourselves as consumers of health care services—at least at first. If you retain some objectivity as you do phone screening of the doctors, it will help you to ask the necessary questions efficiently. If the doctor passes muster on the "technicalities," you can go on to evaluate her or him in your role as the prospective patient, looking for positive signs of compassion, curiosity, and skill.

Where to begin? If you have been relatively open about your problem with family and friends, you may already have been given the names of specialists. Familiarize yourself with why your friend saw this doctor, what seeing this doctor was like, how your friend was helped. Personal referrals aren't always the best way to find the right specialist, but if you ask some questions, you can decide if you yourself would like to call.

You can call or write to your local county medical society or to local university or teaching hospitals and medical centers. You will be given names of specialists, but you will have no prior evaluation to go by in deciding which ones to contact.

The same advice holds for a voluminous listing of infertility specialists compiled by the American Fertility Society. Going through it may feel like going through the phone book. Still, it is a start. You can write to the American Fertility Society at 2131 Magnolia Avenue, Suite 201, Birmingham, Alabama 35256.

If you want to obtain names of specialists in your area who are highly recommended by knowledgeable infertility patients, then you should call the nearest chapter of the organization RESOLVE and ask for names. You will not have names released to you unless you join the chapter, and that's only fair. For the peace of mind in knowing you're getting a tried-and-true physician, the membership fee is well worth it. The additional membership benefits you'll receive will help you become well-informed, and you'll be assured that you can turn to RESOLVE with any future questions you might have.

Now that you have several names, you can screen them with preliminary phone calls. There is no need for you to make three or four office appointments and pay lots of fees just to discover basic facts about each specialist. These initial questions can be answered on the phone by the physician or (more likely) by an assistant, nurse, or receptionist. If the specialist you are calling is at all busy in the field of infertility, phone inquiries from prospective patients are a normal office routine. Plus, you are getting a sneak preview of what the office staff is like—cooperative and friendly, or curt and intimidating? Since you'll have to interact with your doctor's support staff quite a bit, this is useful information to have.

Start by introducing yourself and explain that you are searching for an appropriate infertility specialist to begin a workup. You can explain how you obtained the doctor's name, and ask the staff member if there is time to answer a few questions. Then, plunge in.

- What is the nature of this doctor's infertility specialty? Is there any particular emphasis?
- What is the doctor's training? How long in this practice?
- What is the doctor's hospital affiliation? Are diagnostic facilities used at that hospital? Labs? Is the hospital located near the doctor's practice?
- Does the doctor perform surgeries related to infertility? Are they documented on videotape? Is the doctor trained in microsurgery or laser surgery?
- Is the practice limited to infertility? Does the doctor have an obstetrical practice? If so, are the hours separated?

- How available is the doctor to patients on weekends, days off, holidays?
- If this is a group practice, do patients see more than one doctor?
- If your focus is primarily on the woman's case, how will the man be examined and evaluated?
- What are the standard costs for: office visits, off-hours appointments, pelvic exams, other workup tests? What is the cancellation policy?
- What arrangements for payment do you require? Does the doctor or hospital accept all types of insurance?
- How long is the wait for the first appointment?

If the answers to these questions satisfy you that the practice is qualified and conscientious, you may want to make an appointment for a first visit/consultation. During this office visit, you will continue to evaluate the doctor, but you will also be getting a feel for what it's like to be under this doctor's care. You should be prepared to enlighten the physician about your case as well. As you make the appointment, ask if there are any special instructions for you to follow, and plan for both spouses to attend.

Whether the wait for your appointment is three days or three months, it is now time to get ready to present the doctor with as much useful information as possible, and to inform yourselves so that you won't be thrown by the discussions about infertility that you're going to have.

Learning About Reproduction, Fertility, and Infertility

Reading and learning as much as you can about infertility can transform you. It won't make you pregnant (at least not directly) but it will help you to become a more active patient. You will be able to participate in your workup plans, and be involved and vigilant during any treatment that you may need.

A knowledgeable patient better understands the confusing details that might frustrate and discourage a less well-informed patient. You'll have a general idea of why certain tests have been ordered for you and you'll know how to ask about the results. Knowing what to expect isn't going to scare you away, as some contend, but it will demystify this whole process, which will actually make it less scary.

The ability to follow along with your treatment can help you be a better consumer of your doctor's medical services. You'll be better able to evaluate your physician, and you can begin to understand your doctor's logic in laying out the plans for the workups and treatment. You'll discover that your doctor isn't God and can't wave a magic wand and make you conceive; logical steps must be taken. This is an important realization, because your understanding of your case will make the steps of your workup look like real progress toward your goal—pregnancy.

If you are undergoing a certain treatment over a prolonged period of time, your readings and questions will help you to know when it might be time to try something else. You and your doctor will be able to come to an understanding about what you can do next.

Physicians have started to appreciate actively involved patients. Ask any busy infertility specialist—an involved patient can work so much more energetically with the physician, to the benefit of each. If a doctor becomes nervous or defensive when you show informed curiosity about the handling of your case, it could be a warning sign. If it makes you nervous to show what you know during an office visit, you might question staying with this doctor for the duration of your workup. Most specialists will welcome all your questions and comments, and really use you as a partner in your own care. This can give you back some sense of control over your life.

What to read?

There's no need to build up a huge private library of infertility books in order to get to know the subject. But you can only gain by becoming better informed. Plus, it will give you something concrete to do on those days when you feel like you're going to jump out of your skin.

Now, what to read, and where to find it? If you have a large public library, it's a good place to start. You can find books, plus current magazine and newspaper articles giving the most recent information available on infertility. Starting with general books and articles in popular magazines and daily newspapers is a good way to get acquainted with the basics. There will be time enough later to go to more specialized publications should you ever need them. In the meantime, don't let your research get too complicated.

As you look over the books available, bear in mind that while the information on the basic physiology of men and women is correct, the medical treatments recommended and the kinds of tests ordered might be out of date. If a book concerned strictly with the medical aspects of infertility is more than five to ten years old, you can guess that there's more recent information on the subject. To be brought up to date, it's a good idea to try periodicals.

Use the *Readers' Guide to Periodical Literature* for starters. Looking under "infertility" from the most recent guides to back issues will give you the names of magazines publishing articles on the subject. Look for articles in news magazines and health and fitness magazines as well as in "women's" magazines ... one or two have even appeared in magazines for men. While information found in popular magazines may be somewhat simplified, it will help you find the latest news of developments in the field. Later on, if you need to, try university or medical libraries for the specific periodicals on infertility doctors read.

RESOLVE, Inc., offers a very complete selection of articles, fact sheets, and some books to answer a variety of questions on this subject. Call your local chapter, or write to their national office (RESOLVE, 5 Water Street, Arlington, MA 02174) and ask for a list of publications that can be ordered. Not only can these readings answer most of your medical questions, but they also address the emotional impact of infertility, too. That's something that is generally given short shrift in the medically oriented books.

Home Remedies for Infertility

You're going to run across various home remedies for infertility. You may want to try some of them if they're harmless and you feel that you just have to do something. But bear in mind that the best way to handle your infertility problem is to listen to your doctors, not to your friends. Here are a few of the home cures you'll probably hear about:

After intercourse, stand on your head.

How uncomfortable can you get! Who is in the mood for gymnastics after intercourse? The theory is, of course, to tip your body so that the sperm will drain downward through the cervix, through the uterus, and dribble into the fallopian tubes. Presto, pregnancy.

If you do want the reassurance that you aren't losing any seminal fluid after intercourse, you don't have to stand on your head. Lie on your back, prop a pillow under your rear, stay in bed for twenty to thirty minutes following intercourse, and you'll get equal benefit. If conditions are right for conception, sperm can make a good head start in this time. Remember, healthy sperm will swim all by themselves to their rendezvous, so you don't have to slosh yourself about to achieve the same result. Staying in bed an extra twenty minutes with your partner sounds nicer anyway, doesn't it?

Have sex in the missionary position only.

In normally fertile couples, position for intercourse won't make much difference. But since you are trying, it's a good idea to arrange for the semen to be deposited in the optimum place in the vagina, next to the cervix. The missionary position (distasteful name!), in which the man and woman face one another with the man above, often accomplishes this. It's even better to place a pillow beneath the woman's hips to tilt her pelvis up slightly. Remain lying down (see previous item) for thirty minutes or so before getting up. Keep in mind, though, that it's important to keep your intimate relationship as stress-free as possible, so don't force yourselves into a routine of using only this position.

The woman should drink cough syrup.

Over-the-counter expectorant cough syrups containing the ingredient guaifenesin may thin the consistency or appear to increase the amount of the woman's cervical mucus. While thinning and loosening the nasal mucus to relieve cold symptoms, these syrups sometimes also have the side effect of making the cervical mucus thinner or more copious. Your doctor will probably examine your cervical mucus early on, and let you know if there's a problem, but in the meantime, some people recommend the guaifenesin. Taking any medicine, even over-the-counter ones, is something to avoid, but what if it works . . . ? If you think your mucus is scanty, call your doctor first and ask before you give it a try.

The man should wear boxer shorts.

Men with a lower sperm count should be at the urologist's, not at the department store buying new underwear. Only the doctor can determine if overly warm testes are contributing to infertility. It can't hurt you to try a new style of underwear, but don't let that be the only thing you do. Have several properly spaced semen analyses—there's no substitute for them.

Be sure the woman always has an orgasm.

Physiologically speaking, women do not need to reach orgasm to successfully conceive. If the sperm is deposited in the best spot in the vagina near the cervix, and physical and hormonal factors are favorable, a woman's orgasm is technically icing on the cake. There is some speculation that the muscle contraction of a woman's orgasm after ejaculation might help sperm arrive at their destination just that much sooner, but there are no studies to support this. If your sex life is a little raggy now, don't add this imperative to the pressure. Of course, to keep baby-making sex as nice as possible, it's very important to consider the pleasure of both partners.

Have sex every day in the middle of the month.

You may feel that to hit the right day of ovulation, you should have sex every day in the middle of the woman's cycle. This actually can be counterproductive, in that you could be depleting the man's sperm supply faster than his body can replenish it. Talk to your doctors and hear their recommendations on frequency. Monitoring the woman's cycle with urine tests from the drugstore or watching for the post-ovulatory temperature rise that marks the end of "necessary sex" are ways to avoid frantic hit-or-miss sex. Planning on an every-other-day schedule in the middle of the cycle can also help take the pressure off.

Reviewing Your Medical History

While you await your first appointment with an infertility specialist, you can think about, gather, and record important information on your medical histories. Medical histories are essential in an infertility investigation. They help the doctor tailor your workups to suit your needs, and histories can provide valuable clues. Writing down the details to give the doctor will help in two ways. It's amazing how facts can be forgotten or garbled if you are nervous or distracted during your first visit to the doctor. Writing down what you remember now, while you have more time to think, can keep the facts straight. Also, if you are ever sent to another physician, or need a second opinion, you'll have consistent information going to every doctor.

The medical history questions here aren't the only ones you will be asked. But they do give information that most specialists will need from the start of the workup. There are more questions here for the woman than for the man. It doesn't seem fair! But the reproductive mechanisms in women are more complex and more must be investigated. The study of male infertility is starting to catch up, however, so be prepared to also hear more questions for the man than you see here. Jot them down with your answers to keep for reference, too. Don't be shy about asking why a question has been asked. Your understanding of your case will be enhanced, and you'll see inside the mind of your doctor.

Don't be threatened by questions that seem too personal. It's hard to hear details of your health and personal life reduced to facts on a page, but it does help you to be more objective about discussing them. Also, you may be interviewed separately for a few moments, in case there are details you feel you cannot discuss in front of your partner. It is important to realize that if you have these kinds of secrets from your partner, they may come out anyway during the course of an infertility workup. Giving your doctor separate confidences is certainly not wrong, yet you are placing an extra burden on someone who's trying to help you both. Working out an honest relationship together may be the answer instead.

NOTES FOR FEMALE MEDICAL HISTORY

Menstrual History

Age of first period _____

Character of early periods: erratic, cramps, flow, number of days _____

_____

Did your periods stabilize within a reasonable amount of time?

_____

Do you remember anything unusual about your periods in the past?

_____

Your Periods Today

Do you menstruate regularly? _____

Length of average period, and of entire cycle _____

If you do not menstruate regularly, last period you had was when, and what was it like?

_____

If you are usually regular, have you had any missed periods?

_____

Character of your usual periods, cramps, flow, clotting, etc.

_____

Do you have any premenstrual symptoms? _____

History of Birth Control Use

What methods have you used? When did you use them, for how long? Why did you discontinue using them?

_____

What were your cycles like while using these methods of birth control? What were they like after you stopped using them?

_____

How was your general health while using these birth control methods?

_____

Have you ever been pregnant? Do you have any living children?

_____

Have you had any miscarriages? _____

When was the age of first intercourse? _____

Have you had any sexually transmitted diseases? Which ones, when, and how were they discovered and treated?

_____

Have you ever had a therapeutic abortion? What age? Did you heal without complications?

_____

_____

General Medical Questions

Did your mother take the drug DES while she was pregnant with you?

_____

Have you had any surgeries/hospitalizations? When? Why?

_____

Have you had any chronic illness, now or in childhood?

_____

Have you ever been on medication for a protracted period of time?
Taking any now?

_____

Any infections? _____

How is your gynecological health? Vaginal infections, diseases, abnormal Pap smears?
_____

Are there any chronic conditions or diseases in your family?
_____

Lifestyle Questions

What is your occupation? Are you exposed to any chemicals or radiation on the job?
_____

Do you use any recreational drugs? _____
Are you a long-distance runner or exercise heavily? _____
Does your weight fluctuate much? Are you a dieter? _____
Any history of eating disorders? _____
Do you consider yourself under a lot of stress on the job or at home?
_____

Do you drink alcohol or smoke cigarettes? _____

NOTES FOR MALE MEDICAL HISTORY

About the Reproductive Organs

Have you ever sustained a blow to the scrotum? _____
Have you had the mumps? When? _____
Have you ever had pain in the testicles? Swelling?
_____

Have you ever had a semen analysis? Are the results available?
_____

What was the age of first intercourse? _____
Have you ever had any sexually transmitted diseases?
_____

Have you impregnated any women (including present spouse) in the past?
_____

Have you ever had any problems with impotence?

General Health

Did your mother take the drug DES while she was pregnant with you?

Have you had any surgeries, hospitalizations? When, why?

What illnesses have you had, in childhood, and in adulthood?

Any chronic illnesses?

Have you ever taken any medication for a protracted period of time?

Lifestyle Questions

What is your occupation? Do you have contact with chemicals or radiation on the job? Are you exposed to excessive heat? Do you sit all day?

Do you smoke cigarettes? Marijuana? Do you use alcohol?

Do you use any other recreational drugs? _____

Questions for Both Partners

The doctor will probably ask you about your sexual relationship, frequency of intercourse, and if you are having any problems related to making love. While this is very personal information, and you may feel embarrassed talking about it, try to remember that you're talking to a doctor and this doctor has heard it all before. The doctor will not be shocked, embarrassed, or judge you in any way! Every effort should be made to help you feel comfortable while discussing this subject. Take a deep breath, and remember you're doing this for a good cause.

Start Your Temperature Charts

Even before you see the infertility specialist, you can begin keeping temperature charts. Measuring and recording the woman's basal body temperature (BBT) each morning is a well-known ritual, and sometimes we hope that the making of these charts alone will somehow lead directly to pregnancy. Understanding what the charts really show and how they are interpreted will help you keep this routine in proper perspective.

Most infertility specialists like to have two to three months of temperature charts to interpret for signs that a woman is ovulating. Starting these charts before your appointment, especially if the appointment isn't scheduled for a while, will increase the efficiency of the early stages of your workup since you won't have to wait three more months after you finally see the doctor in order to see what's up with your temperature. Plus, this will give you something positive to do while you wait to get in.

The hormone changes that occur through a woman's monthly cycle are reflected by fluctuations in her body temperature. These changes are so subtle that they are measured in tenths of a degree and thus are only apparent if the temperature is taken when the body has been at rest for at least several hours. That's why you take it first thing in the morning after you wake up, even before you move around or get out of bed.

What BBTs Show and Don't Show

As you begin to fill out your first month's chart of readings, you will see if the temperature line is flat or rises at about the middle of the cycle. These changes usually correspond to the body's hormonal activity.

As the monthly cycle begins with Day 1 of the menstrual period, the temperature may seem erratic. This reflects a fluctuation in the body's hormones during menstruation. As your period ends, the temperature should become more stable. It won't be exactly the same every day, but the readings will be close. During the first half of your cycle, the hormone FSH (follicle-stimulating hormone) is working on your ovaries to produce the monthly egg. During this phase, your temperature should be stable and under about 97.6 degrees Fahrenheit.

As the follicle prepares to release its egg, the hormone balance changes. The output of LH (luteinizing hormone) increases, signalling the ovary to release an egg. This is often called the LH "surge." Ovulation occurs when the egg is released. The corpus luteum (the ruptured egg sac on the ovary) begins to manufacture more of the hormone progesterone, which keeps the uterine lining lush, wet, and ready to receive a fertilized egg.

When the progesterone level rises, a woman's basal body temperature rises, too. The temperature elevation should be well above the temperature before ovulation, usually up one full degree or so. The progesterone level will go up only if a ruptured egg follicle produces progesterone, so the temperature rise indicates ovulation in a normal woman. So, these temperature charts show very generally whether ovulation has occurred or not. What these charts do not do is predict ovulation. Making love strictly by the dictates of the charts probably will not work—it's hindsight, not foresight!

Keep these charts as supplemental information for your infertility specialist. If more specific information about your hormone levels or ovulation is wanted, other tests will be made. Still, the charts are a helpful preliminary tool if they show a distinct temperature rise and reveal a distinct bi-phasic (two levels of temperature) cycle.

Types of Thermometers

There are special basal-temperature mercury thermometers that you can buy at the drugstore. They're similar to the glass thermometers you are used to seeing, except the degree range is very limited and is divided into tenths of a degree. The battery-powered digital thermometers automatically measure temperature in tenths of degrees and are a lot easier to read. Unless you receive specific instructions to do otherwise, the temperature can be taken orally, so be sure you buy an oral thermometer.

Types of Temperature Charts

There are several styles of temperature-chart blanks available, and each has its merits. But when half-asleep early in the morning, things should be kept as simple as possible. With graph-paper styles, it's too difficult to follow the closely spaced lines over to the proper temperature and day axis and draw a dot. It's easier to just circle the numerical reading as it is read from the thermometer. If you faithfully record the proper calendar date for the first day of your cycle, you need not run all the way down the chart, filling them in on each line. Watch for your distinct temperature rise, usually mid-cycle, and date this day and backdate the last day as your next period begins, ending this cycle. (If you like, you can fill in the rest of the dates while waiting to see the doctor. If the first day is dated correctly, just chant, "Thirty days hath September," and write.)

How to Take and Record Basal Body Temperature

The BBT is the temperature of the body after at least several hours of rest. This fact is repeated here because understanding it makes the strange routine explained here seem less strange!

1. The first day you get your menstrual period is the first day of your new cycle. Fill in the date on the top date blank, opposite "Day 1." Get a pencil or pen, and put the chart and the pen somewhere near your bed. The thermometer must be placed within your reach while you are lying in bed, since you're going to be grabbing it right after you awaken. Don't worry if you missed taking your temperature on Day 1 or even on Day 2 or Day 3 of your period. Write "period" over the temperature numerals, and leave it at that.

2. You must start recording your temperature by Day 4. The night before you begin your readings you must shake down a mercury thermometer, if that's what you're using. If you do this in the morning, the basal reading will be lost. If you use a digital thermometer, check the battery to make sure it's working. Put the thermometer within easy reach so you can get to it even if you are half-asleep.

3. When you first awaken, don't stir, just quietly reach for the thermometer and position it correctly in your mouth. Lie quietly for a full five minutes (mercury) or until the thermometer beeps (digital). If your mornings are chaotic, featuring pets jumping on your head or other distractions, plan ahead. Set your alarm slightly earlier or have your partner keep the peace.

4. You need not immediately record the temperature reading if you're using a mercury thermometer. Take it out of your mouth, and lay it down very gently in a protected, padded spot on the night table. The reading won't change until the thermometer is shaken down. If you're not getting out of bed right away, or if you're forgetful, knowing this helps! When you're more fully awake, you can better read and accurately record the temperature. Right after you record the reading, get in the habit of shaking down the thermometer for the next day. Or

if you can remember, you can record, shake down, and replace the thermometer right before you go to sleep that night.

Some digitals retain the reading for a long period. Does yours? Test it first. You can't put the thermometer aside and go back to sleep if the reading will be lost. Some digitals are hard to read in the dim light of early morning. How is yours? Overall, it is best to read and record a digitally measured temperature right after you take it, to avoid losing the reading or wearing down the battery.

5. When you record the reading, just circle the proper numbers on the chart line that corresponds to your cycle day. The rest of the space on the line is used to record pertinent details about the reading, including your health, sleep disruption, stress, and use of alcohol the night before. All of these things can affect the reading. Write in "took temperature late," "have the flu," "overslept," or anything else that changes the good night's rest you normally have.

6. Your doctor will be interested in seeing your patterns of sexual intercourse during the month, so try to remember to put an "X," a check mark, or a "C" (for coitus) on the days when you make love. Don't jump out of bed, leaving your partner, to fill in a check mark! Just try to remember to fill it in the next day.

7. Don't get into a pattern of achievement anxiety with your temperatures or with filling in your intercourse habits. This is just a chart, a piece of paper that can provide some general information for your doctor. If you forget once or twice, write in that you forgot. Don't fudge a reading, though we all have been tempted to do so at times! The very fact that you are forgetting a lot or haven't had intercourse much is also information—about the level of stress in your life. The doctor needs to know that, too.

8. Both partners can participate in taking and recording the temperatures. It takes pressure off the woman and gives the man a chance to feel more involved. Plus, if your doctor later instructs you to watch your chart as you make love through the middle of the cycle, the woman won't feel as though she's dictating the schedule of lovemaking.

9. Don't use temperature charts as a bargaining chip with fate. You may feel that you're paying your dues now, so you deserve a pregnancy

even more. Remember that these charts are a rough diagnostic tool, and that doctors have different theories on how to interpret them. Charts don't carry a magic within them to make you pregnant; their information only becomes useful after your doctor has seen them and explained to you what they show.

Taking temperatures can be an adventure at first. It's fascinating to participate in a "scientific" data-gathering activity to help find out how to help you conceive, and you'll like the feeling of doing something worthwhile. The secret to temperature taking is that even after the novelty wears off, you've got to keep it up. Every specialist has a philosophy on how much temperature information is needed, so be sure that when you go for your appointment, you find out how long you'll have to keep track. After a while, you may even find that the habit becomes hard to break.

Thoughts About Taking Your Temperature

Dorothy Hagerty

At first it was a real challenge to be diligent enough to remember every morning. Then you were taking your temperature and didn't even realize it—it became instinct. And how about the mornings you forgot? Did you cheat a little and put a temperature down anyway? Of course you did. Or have you awakened, put the thermometer into your mouth, then fallen back to sleep? When you woke up, the thermometer was gone, right? (I lost a thermometer once in the water bed, and didn't find it again until we moved!) Or, how do you explain the thermometer when you're spending the night at someone else's house, especially at grandmother's!

Taking my temperature became a game for me. It was a real challenge to see how long I could go before I screwed up. I was not about to let temperature taking run my life! I was going to run my life! I laugh about it, and when I get discouraged I think how silly I must look lying in bed with this thing in my mouth.

But at least I have a good reason to keep taking my temperature. This gives me the hope and inspiration to continue doing it.

Using Urine Testing Kits to Watch for Ovulation

Urine testing kits, bought at the drugstore without prescription and used at home, are a godsend. These kits provide information on ovulation that was once only available from a doctor. At home, in private, you can monitor your urine for traces of your LH (luteinizing hormone) surge, which triggers egg release. You can plan to make love accordingly. The kits help you to figure out the time of optimum fertility before you've even been to the doctor's. And you will know about ovulation *before* it occurs, not after, as is the case with temperature charts.

If you think you have a fertility problem, using a urine test kit at home is no substitute for proper medical attention. But using one before seeing a specialist might yield useful information, and it will certainly help acquaint you with the workings of your body. It also helps give you back some control over your life.

By all means, try using a kit for a month or two, plan intercourse, and see how you do. If used correctly, it can help you hit the right day, which could result in pregnancy. Even if no pregnancy results, it will start to settle the question if you are ovulating or not.

When you first begin using these tests, you may see yourself back in a high school chemistry class. There are several chemical reactions that must be timed accurately, which result in a final color change. This color change signals the presence of LH in a larger amount than usual. That's your LH surge, which should trigger ovulation.

To catch the pronounced difference in LH amount, you must start testing your urine *before* you think you'll be ovulating. You have to think about the general character of your past cycles in terms of their length and figure out when to start testing. The kits tell you how to do this.

Read all the instructions before you start any testing. It sounds too obvious to mention here, but these tests are tricky, and you have to know what you're doing before you try. Don't stand over the bathroom sink, holding a cup of urine, reading about what to do next! If you're still sleepy and you're collecting your first urination of the day, this is doubly important.

Follow the instructions with absolute dedication to accuracy. Use a reliable kitchen timer—or a calculator, or a digital watch that has a stopwatch-type timer. Save the extra urine you may have left over, in case you need to repeat the test. When you're finished, you can safely dispose of all liquids in the toilet.

If you'd like to share the responsibility for monitoring cycles, the test can be performed by your partner, who will then record the results. You'll both feel vitally involved.

The kits are reasonably priced, but they could become expensive if you use them every month indefinitely. Ask your specialist about continuing to use them once you are officially under the doctor's care. You may be asked to use one to time your postcoital test, and perhaps again later to time intercourse or for inseminations, so you'll already be familiar with how they work.

Watching for Changes in Cervical Mucus

If a woman is very observant of body signs, she can learn to look for changes in her cervical mucus that could help indicate ovulation.

Through the first ten to twelve days of her cycle, a woman's cervix gradually produces more mucus, and the mucus itself changes in consistency. It is initially cloudy and tacky, but as ovulation draws nearer, the mucus becomes clear, thin, and slippery. This clear, copious, and slippery mucus is designed to assist the sperm in swimming up through the cervix and beyond, to find the newly emerging egg. When ovulation has occurred and sperm assistance is no longer needed, the cervical mucus changes again, becoming thicker, more cloudy and tacky. The vagina feels dry by the end of the cycle, when this pattern starts again.

The changes in your mucus can be observed by checking your vaginal secretions with a clean finger. When thin, clear mucus appears during your cycle, you might also feel the sensation of wetness and see the "egg white" mucus on toilet tissue or on your underpants. You may feel that you're "drying up" a few days later, as secretions lessen and change back to a thicker consistency.

If you observe "egg whites," you might well interpret this as a sign that ovulation mechanisms are working, but only more sophisticated testing can tell for sure. As you see this thin, clear mucus, check with a urine test kit, and see if your temperature chart indicates a rise in a day or so. You might be well on the way to pinpointing ovulation on your own. Tell your doctor what you have observed and ask about the best way to use this information as you try to conceive.

Mittelschmerz

You may have heard that some women can "feel" themselves ovulating. This is probably a reference to mittelschmerz, a German word meaning "middle pain."

It is theorized that the release of hormones and blood from the ovulating ovary, or the movement of the fimbria end of the fallopian tube, could cause a twinge of slight pain felt on the corresponding side of the abdomen. This discomfort could be momentary or last several hours. This sensation, felt in the middle of the cycle, is mittelschmerz.

It's intriguing to think that all women can actually feel themselves ovulating, but this isn't so. Not many women actually feel mittelschmerz and it alone is a poor indicator of ovulation. When you go to your doctor, certainly report it if you feel such a twinge in the middle of your cycle, but don't sit around "listening" to your body in hopes of picking up the signal. That pain you're so sure is mittelschmerz could really be last night's pizza. So, keep your energies focused on the more positive, tangible activities you can do right now. If you do feel mittelschmerz, consider it a bonus, not an essential.

Making Love by the Calendar

Up to this point in your life, making love has been an experience prompted by romantic urges. Any couple has its own patterns of sexual communication that develop as the relationship develops. Seldom has any outside influence interfered with what most of us consider the most natural and pleasurable side of commitment.

Making love according to the dictates of the woman's monthly cycle, something infertile couples often must do in order to conceive, can really come as a shock. It can damage spontaneity, for starters. It can change making love from an expression of love and passion to an exercise in self-consciousness. In the extreme, it can make couples dread going into their bedrooms. When ovulation seems imminent, the pressure to perform intensifies.

While these complications of your love life sound ominous, they don't all happen to everyone in the extreme. But unless you're made of stone, you'll feel some of this pressure. If you don't like making love by the calendar, you are not alone!

Two imperatives are clashing here: getting pregnant and preserving and nurturing a loving, open sexual relationship. Together you must work out a balance between these two objectives.

Right now, achieving pregnancy is probably uppermost in your minds. For the time being, certain sacrifices in the romance department are certainly worth it. And for most couples, their sexual relationship will settle down again after the months of trying are past. So right now a full-out effort to hit the right day seems in order.

If you do decide to go in this direction, don't neglect your relationship. This is a stressful time for you, even if you are both fully enthusiastic for a pregnancy ASAP. Be extra good to each other. Go out on "dates." Dote on each other. Soothe each other after a rough day at work. Make extra time for each other, and really listen as you talk together about your feelings, hopes, and fears. Avoid situations that make you tense. Count to ten rather than have a petty argument. Really put in the effort, even if you think you don't need to! It's money in the bank for your relationship.

If you are experiencing tension because of this pressure, recognize that this is a problem every couple must deal with along with infertility. It just goes with the territory. There's a myth that couples fighting infertility are of one mind, always agreeing, always miserable together, always happy together, soldiering on to conceive their baby. Not true! You are two distinct individuals in the other areas of your lives, and it's no different with infertility. You will hit some bumps, you will disagree. That's why you should give yourself as many breaks as you can. Keep talking, keep joking, keep kissing. Use facts to dispel fears. Don't assign blame. Try to put yourself in your partner's place and empathize. Have patience, patience, patience. There's always next month!

As your doctor begins to help you work out your infertility problems in the months ahead, you can shift some of the burden of initiative from your shoulders to hers. If you trust your doctor, you can ask for help in working out just how necessary this obligatory lovemaking might be in your particular case. Taking a break every few months wouldn't be so terrible either, if you feel you still have plenty of time to try. Ask and find out. Let your physician know that you want to have a baby, and you want to achieve it within a healthy and warm sexual relationship. Your physician will treat you that much more compassionately, and some of your apprehensions about this whole baby-making business will disappear.

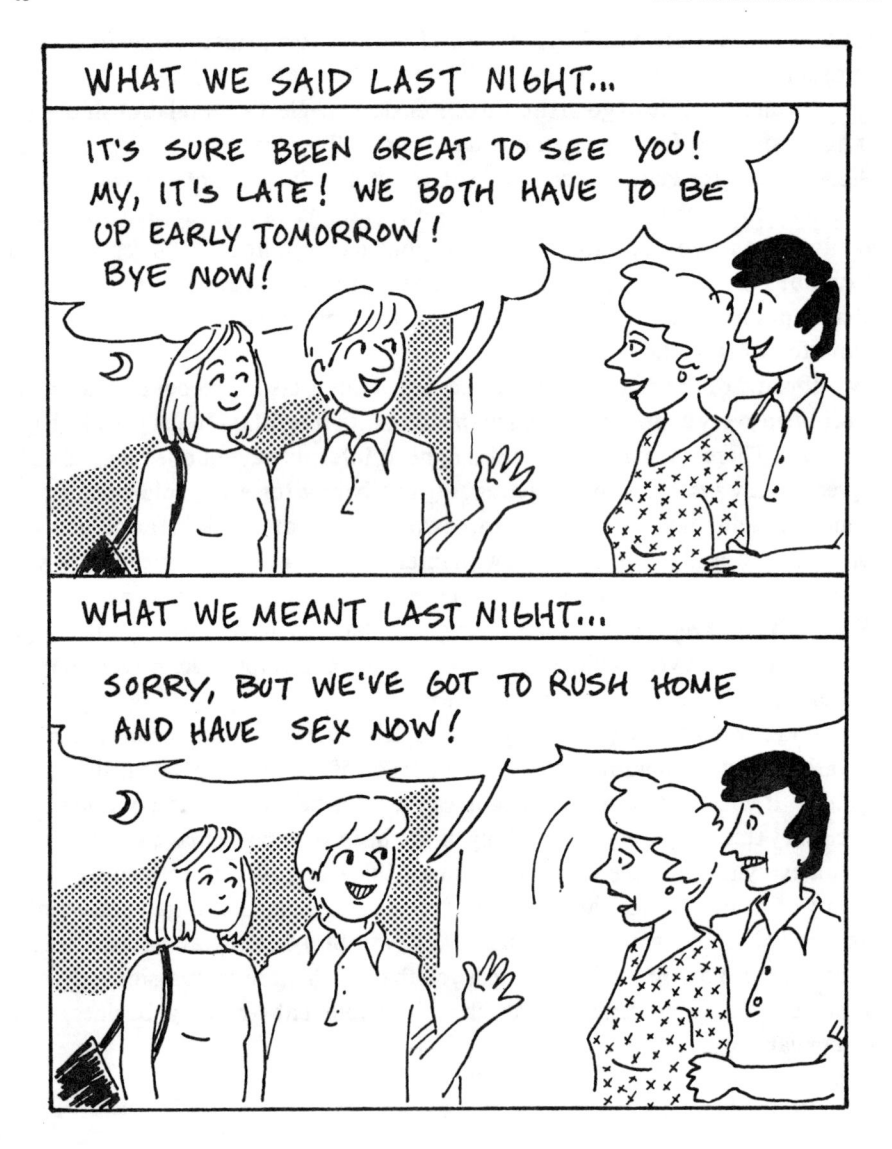

THE INFERTILITY MAZE

WHAT WE SAID LAST NIGHT...

IT'S SURE BEEN GREAT TO SEE YOU! MY, IT'S LATE! WE BOTH HAVE TO BE UP EARLY TOMORROW! BYE NOW!

WHAT WE MEANT LAST NIGHT...

SORRY, BUT WE'VE GOT TO RUSH HOME AND HAVE SEX NOW!

SECTION II

Your Infertility Is Investigated: The Workups

Section II will help you to work with your doctor to discover problems that could be hampering your fertility.

You can read here about how to evaluate your infertility specialist as you go in for your first appointment. Then, the tests of the infertility workups for both men and women will be described, so that you can discuss them fully with the doctor.

Importantly, you will also find that this section includes pages where both of you can record the results of your tests for future reference. This will help you to form the best picture of your condition that you can, and it will give you access to these results later, when you may have questions or problems. If you want to read further about a test or a condition, knowing your own results will help you understand what's happening. Plus, if you ever want an informal second opinion, you will have accurate information for other medical professionals to consider.

Read through the table of contents for this section, and you'll see that there is special advice on coping with the inconveniences that infertility testing can cause. In addition, it is important that at this stressful time communication between partners not be neglected. It's natural to want the most efficient investigation possible, but you should not rush into it at the expense of your personal relationship. Reading this section will remind you to take this experience step by step, and to always stop along the way to talk and listen to one another.

As Your Appointment Approaches, How Are You Feeling?

As your first appointment with an infertility specialist draws near, you'll probably experience some strong emotions. Going in to start an evaluation is an important step forward, but even if you feel relieved about it, you may also be nervous, impatient, apprehensive. This is normal.

If you feel nervous about your first meeting with the doctor, try to be as prepared as you can for it. Write down your questions so you won't forget to ask them. Go over your medical histories and do some reading so you'll be better able to understand the language of the discussion. If you feel ready for this meeting, you might also feel calmer.

You may be apprehensive. Most of this fear comes from the realization that you are about to face something unknown. What will the doctor be like? What will the doctor do to us? What will be found? Will we be helped?

It's true that you won't discover what the doctor is like until you have your appointment. But if you found your specialist through a reliable recommendation, you probably already have some information. Dealing with the staff over the telephone can also give you a clue about the atmosphere around the office. Plus you know that during the appointment you have questions to ask, an evaluation of your own to make.

If one of your concerns is what the doctor will "do to us," remember this very important fact: you do have control over your tests and treatments. The doctor isn't going to order any tests against your will; nothing will be done without your understanding and consent. You and the doctor will be working together as a team every step of the way. If you ask questions, inform yourselves, and participate mentally in your workup processes, you will avoid feeling like a guinea pig.

Fearing what the doctor will find over the course of this workup is a very natural emotion. It isn't a fear that can be eliminated with a few instructions, for this is the central problem you face now: is something wrong?

How you deal with this unknown is probably going to be similar to how you handled comparable situations in the past. Think of your first day of high school, a big job interview, moving to a new town. Were you worried or curious? Optimistic to learn new things? Ready to face a challenge? These past experiences, while somewhat daunting at the time, did work out. Bearing this in mind will put your newest challenge into perspective.

Granted, the unknown you face now probably seems like one of the most important you've ever had to consider. Concentrating on the process of solving this unknown, rather than fearing the results, can give you some room to breathe. You will be working with your doctor's expertise to run tests and pick up clues. These are positive steps toward ending this riddle of infertility. You may fear the diagnosis may be complicated, but there's also an excellent chance statistically that your problem is simple and pretty easy to treat. But you won't know until you have started your workups.

Do you feel impatient to get this show on the road? This isn't a surprising reaction, especially if you've had to wait a while to get your appointment. Don't resent the doctor for this waiting period—it gave you a chance to get used to the whole idea of the infertility workup, to become mentally ready. This wait won't be characteristic of all your appointments, either. A good doctor will assure you that you will be seen promptly, on the day you need to be seen, from now on.

Don't let your impatience rush you into too many tests too soon. If you're very anxious to get started quickly, explain this concern to your doctor as you discuss your case. The doctor will plan your workup with a timetable that takes your needs into account, but that has your medical priorities in mind, too.

Do you feel a bit sad about seeing an infertility specialist? If you do, you're not alone. Everyone who has had even a minor problem with infertility has felt let down about it. You are entitled to react to this situation appropriately: it is sad that this had to happen to your plans for a family right now. Don't kick yourself if you're not thrilled to be doing this.

You may even feel depressed and discouraged about needing medical attention for a fertility problem. Going in for your appointment could make you feel branded with a scarlet "I." You may hope nobody you know sees you going into the doctor's office. You may feel disbelief that this is really happening to you. These are common, very human, feelings.

One thing you can do is to think of this appointment not as the end, but as a beginning. That's really what it is. Both of you are seeking out the help you need, which is the right thing to do. You're beginning a search for the answer that has up to now eluded you. You are starting an important relationship with a medical professional that could end up bringing you great happiness. These are positive steps to feel good about.

Talking Together About Your Expectations

It's important to make every effort to go together to this first appointment with the infertility specialist. The feeling that you are sharing this experience will alleviate some of the jitters, and besides, you're both vitally involved anyway.

Before you go to the doctor's, talk together about what you each think and feel about taking this step. Each of you should try to be supportive of the other's reaction to this event, and you each should acknowledge that you will react as individuals to what happens.

You are each used to seeing doctors one-on-one, so having a joint medical appointment will be different. You each will be describing yourself to the doctor, discussing needs, asking questions. Importantly, each of you will be forming your own relationship with the specialist, and the two relationships will differ. Your initial reactions to the doctor may not match, either.

Don't concern yourself with presenting an artificially united front to the doctor or about disagreeing privately about your impressions later. A full discussion of your feelings is essential to finding the right specialist for you. Set aside some time the day following your appointment and talk about your feelings together after you each have had time to think.

The First Appointment: How to Evaluate Your Specialist

Two things will go on at your first meeting. You are there to find a specialist you can work with and whom you trust. Your specialist will want to hear about your situation, and will be thinking about what kind of help you may need. That's a lot of important business for one appointment.

Being alert from the minute you come into the waiting room will help you get the most complete impression of this doctor and the assistants in the office. As you arrive, how are you greeted by the staff? Is the reception area inviting? Are there magazines other than maternity reading on hand? Is there reading material on infertility available?

How long do you have to wait to see the doctor? Is there a restroom handy? Is there a telephone you can use? These may seem like trivial questions, and they aren't the most earth-shattering issues, but if you're going to be visiting this doctor frequently, these small comforts add up.

As you go in to see the doctor, you might be nervous. If you are, just acknowledge it, and comment to the doctor about it to help break the ice. The doctor's reaction to this admission will give you a clue to the kind of "bedside manner" you might expect. Does the doctor hear the comment, reacting to it in a compassionate, reassuring manner? Are your fears brushed aside a little too quickly? Only you can say how much concern you'd like to receive from your doctor.

As you discuss your case, what is the doctor doing? Is she preoccupied, or listening to you carefully? After hearing a key complaint, is your description of your problem cut off before you're finished? Are you given time to fully talk about why you're there?

As the doctor answers your questions, are you being treated as an intelligent person in need of help? If you need an answer more fully explained, is the doctor willing to repeat and expand the reply?

If you like, take a list of questions into the office with you. A good physician will understand and not make you feel self-conscious about reading from notes. If you want to jot something down, by all means, do so.

How does the doctor describe infertility, how it's investigated, how it's treated? Is it discussed as an interesting scientific problem, or as a complex emotional and physiological problem? As the doctor refers to her practice, are any limitations acknowledged? Are you promised a pregnancy, plain and simple? (Beware.) Is the doctor willing to discuss success rates?

Does this doctor know about RESOLVE? Are you encouraged to participate in your local chapter's activities and use its educational materials? This is a good clue that your doctor will be glad to have a well-informed, active patient.

A good infertility specialist recognizes that it's hard to separate the emotional aspects from the medical facts of your case. Ask if there is any referral available should you wish to talk to a counselor at any time while under this doctor's care. You definitely want a physician who takes your emotional well-being into account.

After you've been interviewed jointly, your doctor may ask to see each of you separately for a few minutes. This reassures couples who may each have private information to add to their medical histories. This is just a formality for most couples, and it may even shock you if you've never considered keeping any information from your partner. But it is a reality that an experienced infertility specialist will have handled in the past. If this separate interview is handled with grace and a minimum of embarrassment, you're seeing a diplomat as well as a doctor.

If you need time to think about what you've heard and learned during your consultation, that's fine. If the doctor would like to start your workup with a pelvic exam the same day, it's really up to you to decide if you'd like to begin then. Make an appointment for a date in the very near future and go home and talk it over if you need to. If you don't want to continue with this doctor, you can cancel the appointment. If you're eager to start and you feel comfortable with this physician, you'll be making a head start on the workup.

Questions to Ask the Specialist at the First Appointment

If you're not sure what you need to know or you just need a little prompting to start thinking about your appointment, here are some questions to discuss with your specialist.

1. How did you choose infertility as your specialty? What is your training?
2. Are most of your patients infertility patients?
3. Do you have a special interest within infertility that you concentrate on?
4. Will you treat us as a couple, or refer us to the appropriate doctors?
5. Do you do any testing in the office yourself, or do we go to a hospital or lab?
6. What hospital do you use?
7. Do you have experience administering and monitoring Clomid, Pergonal, or other fertility drugs?
8. Are you trained as a surgeon? Do you use microsurgical techniques when possible? Do you do laser surgery? Can you refer us to a physician who does?
9. Will you document surgeries for our records?
10. Do you see patients on weekends, holidays, evenings, or other off times?
11. Who would I see if you are not available? Will he or she know my case?
12. Can you refer us to a counselor, should we ever want one?

13. How do you feel about psychological counseling in cases of infertility?
14. Will you help us to lay out a plan for testing and treatment so that we will know what to expect?
15. Do you take or return phone calls from patients if we have any questions or problems?
16. Are you familiar with RESOLVE? What is your opinion of this organization?
17. What would you say is your percentage of successes with your infertility patients?
18. Do you deliver babies or do you refer your pregnant patients to an obstetrician?

Talking to Your Doctor

Doctors, even compassionate ones, can sometimes be intimidating figures. Infertility specialists, who are very much in demand, often run very busy offices. When we visit the doctor, we may be conscious of our need for help, and as a result begin to feel vulnerable. We realize that our doctors have the power to help us with our difficulty, and we might transfer to them certain powers they don't really possess. If we've waited a long time for this appointment, we might be grateful even to be seen at all. Once inside the office, we might become afraid we'll ask a stupid question, afraid we might be judged.

These emotional responses to seeing the doctor are common and they can combine to make us more passive as patients than we are in the rest of our lives. If we are hearing upsetting or complex explanations, we can almost feel like a detached spectator, observing our appointment from afar.

Of course you should afford your doctors the respect they deserve, but don't forget that you possess certain rights as a patient and consumer of medical services. Therefore, try to make a special effort to be an alert participant in planning and carrying out your infertility care.

You have the right to have your concerns, no matter how "silly," addressed seriously. No question is silly! You should not feel inhibited from asking questions by your doctor's manner in answering. You should have your doctor's full attention while you're in consultation. You are owed a full and understandable explication of your tests and treatments before you undertake any of them. You can see your records any time you like—they are yours.

Asking for more attention from a busy doctor is hard, especially if you're feeling vulnerable. But you don't have to become defensive or strident. You expect patience from your specialist and the staff, so exercise some yourself if you can. Let the doctor finish the explanation, then slowly but deliberately ask your questions. "Do you have time for a few more questions?" is a polite request you can make that would be hard to refuse.

If you think you'll have trouble remembering test results or instructions, jot notes down in this book or another notebook. Keep all your questions here too, and make your way down your list. Keeping this book with you will also give you something to hold onto if you are feeling nervous.

You may have an urge just to be a good patient and leave it at that. Both you and your doctor want you to be a good patient. But this type of good patient isn't the kind who is very quiet, has no questions, and disappears quickly. A good patient is the type who can be frank and open with the doctor, expects frankness in return, and is willing to participate actively in test and treatment planning. Even if you don't feel like you have the energy to jump into this with both feet, making time to talk to the doctor and ask all your questions will at least help you feel you're getting the most out of your office visits.

The Workup Is Planned

During this first consultation with the infertility specialist, you will be hearing about the tests used to investigate fertility problems. In recent years, the necessity for a certain basic group of tests has been acknowledged and adopted by most doctors who are up to date in this field. These tests can usually uncover the more common causes of infertility and can often provide clues leading to the discovery of more unusual problems.

This core group of tests is commonly referred to as the workup. The tests advised for the woman's workup are more extensive than those for the man, at least in the initial stages. As the tests are recounted to you, don't automatically think the doctor is giving too little notice to male infertility. It's just that more things can go wrong in a woman's reproductive system. Each aspect is given a distinctive test. At the beginning, many of the problems found in men can turn up in a skillfully done semen analysis and physical exam. It's just a fact of life.

The prospect of going through a workup can be intriguing—perhaps the mystery will be solved. Or it can be daunting—at this age, few of us have faced such extensive medical scrutiny. Recognize your range of feelings about the workup, and discuss them together and with the doctor as you plan.

How you feel about your infertility, as opposed to how you feel about facing intensive testing, must be balanced as the timetable of your workups is mapped out. If you are tired of waiting or you feel you are running out of time, you may want to plan an efficient, speedy workup. In fact, if you are over thirty or if you have some unusual factors present in your medical history, your doctor should be more than willing to run your workup with as much speed as the woman's cycles will allow, often within two to three months.

If you choose a rapid workup, beware of two possible problems. You may begin to feel besieged by all the medical attention you're suddenly receiving. It might alter your self-image slightly from that of a well person with a problem to that of a "sickly" person. Plus, if you must pay for testing up front and wait for insurance reimbursement, your wallet will be in for a shock. Some of these tests are expensive. Your eagerness to get started on finding the problem, and support from your partner, should carry you through.

Some doctors, after considering the medical and psychological factors in a particular case, may recommend that the workups be stretched out over three to six months. This can take some of the pressure off and promote a less crisis-oriented atmosphere. If you are in your twenties and you don't yet feel that you're up against a biological deadline, you might prefer to have the testing stretched out a bit. It can be a comfort to think that perhaps during the months of testing, you could conceive on your own. It happens many times. Another advantage is that you can stretch out your expenses over a longer period of time.

If you choose to be tested over a longer period of time, it's important to be sure the workup is logically planned and thorough. You may lose time if a problem is found many months from now. Using clues from your medical history and through a physical exam, your doctor will have an idea of what should be investigated first. Go for the suspected problems early if you want a longer testing period.

Ultimately, deciding your timetable is up to you. The most efficient workup is timed according to the woman's cycle, which dictates when many of the tests can be most safely performed and reveal the optimum amount of information. Since it doesn't run on a cycle, a man's reproductive system can be tested at any given point while the woman's tests are in progress. Most basic workups can be completed in two to three months, with the most time-crunched ones coming in at four to six weeks. Find out what your individual timetables might be, and how much running around you'll have to do in getting to various labs, diagnostic centers, hospitals. How will you pay for these tests, and will your insurance reimburse? Is there a chance you'll need to arrange time off from your job? Take as many factors into your planning as possible, and surprises, inconveniences, and lost time will be minimized.

Overview of the Workup: Women

Here is a chart breaking down the basic tests that usually comprise the woman's workup. As you read bear in mind that every workup is going to be different because every patient is different. So your tests might be given in an order unlike what you see here. In fact, you may not need all these tests. You should know why certain tests have been ordered and why certain ones are ruled out, so be sure you understand the reasoning behind your own workup. You and your specialist don't want to overlook any of the common causes of female infertility, nor do you want the earliest findings to halt your investigation until you both have a complete picture of your reproductive health.

Generally, the woman's workup starts with the "noninvasive" tests—that is, the tests that don't require any surgical procedures. The more complex tests are delayed until they are absolutely necessary or as your doctor suggests. If you are having a workup over a very short period of time, your cycle will determine when certain tests can be made, so the order may change for this reason, too.

Whether your workup is short or gradual, be sure your partner is being examined concurrently. Both of you should be present should you need any of the more complicated tests, such as the hysterosalpingogram, endometrial biopsy, or laparoscopy. Supporting each other and experiencing the tests together whenever possible will keep you feeling close during this time.

OVERVIEW OF WOMAN'S WORKUP

Name of test or procedure	What the test is looking for	When can it be performed (in an average 28-day cycle)	Pain?
medical history	past clues to infertility problem	first appt.	no
physical exam	general health and signs of fertility problems	at first appt. or at a subsequent appt.	no
pelvic exam	shape, position of reproductive organs, examine cervix, mucus, assess general reproductive health	not during period	no
blood tests	assay hormone and general health	when needed	pinpricks
urine test	general health	at physical	no
temperature charts	length of cycles, signs of ovulation, record of sexual activity	take temps at home in mornings	no
postcoital or Sims-Huhner test	quality of cervical mucus, ability of sperm to penetrate it, approx. sperm count, signs of (sexually transmitted diseases) or bacteria	near time of ovulation, days 12 to 14 (approx.)	no: feels the same as a pelvic exam

Name of test or procedure	What the test is looking for	When can it be performed (in an average 28-day cycle)	Pain?
endometrial biopsy	check uterine lining and progesterone levels	after day 21 (be sure there is no pregnancy)	some pain and cramping, but it's over very quickly
hysterosalpingogram	fallopian tube patency, shape of inner uterus	early in cycle, days 7 to 10	some pain or cramping
diagnostic laparoscopy	abdominal adhesions, signs of endometriosis, scar tissue, tubal damage	after ovulation in most cases, sometimes before ovulation	small incision made, general anesthesia used. Gas pumped into abdomen may cause discomfort afterwards
ultrasound (optional)	egg development uterine examination	depends on reason for the procedure	no, but a full bladder is often required

Overview of the Workup: Men

As you look at the test list for men, you may be startled at the much lower number of tests given compared to those given to the woman. This does not mean that infertility problems are overwhelmingly found in the woman—untrue. In fact, men and women equally share the problems that cause infertility. The statistics usually report that about 33 percent of causes are found in women alone, 33 percent in men alone, and about 20 percent are shared problems which result in infertility. The remaining causes, about 14 percent, are unknown.

There are more factors present in the female reproductive system that must be evaluated separately, hence more tests. However, the male role in infertility is complex, too. The difference is that these complexities can usually be analyzed by a number of tests done on the man's semen sample. One semen analysis can reveal much important information and yield clues for more comprehensive testing if it is needed.

The man may visit a urologist, as recommended by his primary infertility specialist. At this first visit, be prepared to repeat (with consistency) details of

OVERVIEW OF THE MAN'S WORKUP

Name of test or procedure	What the test is looking for	When can it be performed?	Pain?
medical history	past clues to infertility and lifestyle factors in infertility	office visit	no
physical exam	general health; clues to infertility-related conditions	first appt. or at visit to specialist	no
semen analysis	sperm count; sperm quality; seminal fluid; infections, antibodies	schedule several as directed by specialist	no

your medical, sexual, and lifestyle histories. This specialist may have some brand new questions to ask you, too. Make a note of any new information you uncover that your other doctor will want to know as well.

After a physical exam and histories are noted, the main focus will turn to semen analyses. There should be plans to have two or three of them, spread out over the course of the woman's workup, and at least several weeks apart. Be sure you understand the doctor's instructions for providing the samples, which includes how long to abstain from sex prior to giving the samples and how much time should elapse between analyses.

While semen testing may seem quite nonthreatening to a woman who is undergoing, say, exploratory surgery, it usually is no picnic for the man. Understanding the delicate nature of this test is essential. The prospect of providing a specimen in a jar for others to examine can be caunting, and you may dislike even discussing it. But try to keep your feelings out in the open, and acknowledge the frustration and embarrassment. The awkwardness and stress of infertility testing is not the exclusive property of either partner, so try to have patience, sympathy, and understanding for one another.

Coping with the Inconveniences of the Workups

Schedule Disruption

Expect your work and private schedules to be somewhat chaotic during the weeks of your workups. If you can plan ahead to be more flexible before the crunch comes, you'll experience less stress and strain.

The main disruption will be that the planning of activities will virtually revolve around your monthly cycle. Many of the woman's tests are given only during certain phases of the month, so the calendar will be a fierce dictator. Plus, until Day 1 of each cycle, you'll be uncertain how your next four weeks will be planned. When a new cycle begins, your schedule can be roughly estimated and you'll be able to make plans accordingly.

If you were planning time off for a long weekend or a vacation, this is not the best time to do it unless you are spreading your workup tests over several months. You may find your country inn reservation penciled in for the same Saturday you're suddenly scheduled for a postcoital test. If you save your getaway as a reward after you have completed your workup, you'll have something wonderful to look forward to.

Sex on Schedule

The biggest intrusion you'll have to cope with will be the mechanization of your sex life. You may already have been trying to hit fertile days with your lovemaking, but now you both have to be in the mood according to marching orders given by your doctors, the thermometer, or the results of a home ovulation kit. Perhaps more than once you'll be making love knowing that in a few hours you're having a Sims-Huhner (postcoital) test.

There's little advice that can make these experiences fun, but they don't have to be dreaded, either. Bearing in mind your higher goal (pregnancy) can help you feel positive. And remember, your sex life isn't going to be regulated like this forever. You can look forward to other parts of the month when sex is not for baby making. It's recess! And, you can always take a month or so off from this schedule once your workup is complete. You do have the power to determine the best ways to keep your romantic lives as bright as possible; your doctors don't care what you decide to do on Day 4 or Day 28. Keeping your intimate relationship intact is just as important as achieving a pregnancy. Remind yourselves who was precious to you first—your partner, of course. Cherish each other, even if you're not particularly thrilled to make love at a certain moment. Laugh about it, gripe about it, grin and bear it together.

Job Disruption

During the months of the infertility workups, there probably will be minimum disruption of the man's day-to-day schedule. Since a semen analysis can be planned without worrying about the calendar day, most men can have their physical exams and analyses without having to take time off from the job.

For a woman, however, it's another story. She probably has more tests, and the tests are time-consuming. Unlike a semen specimen that can be dropped off, women have to be there, in the flesh, for their tests.

Doing some planning for one or two days off from work, if you can possibly afford it, will really take the pressure off. You might be able to take a personal day, or you could take a sick or vacation day. For the major tests such as a hysterosalpingogram, it's a must. Even a half-day off (that includes a nice lunch with your partner) can make the postcoital test experience far more pleasant.

Of course, most of us have jobs where this kind of scheduling isn't easy to arrange. It may be too early yet to let the big bosses in on these medical details. Unless you're very sure of their understanding, save your explanations until a later date. After all, these really are only tests. If you feel secure about it, you might take a trusted co-worker into your confidence and try to figure out how to arrange a few hours' absence with the least fuss.

YOUR INFERTILITY IS INVESTIGATED: THE WORKUPS 65

If you enjoy being challenged on the job you may not notice the extra stress that may come during your workup weeks. But if you think that you're going to be given a complicated assignment or be sent on a business trip, you'll have extra arrangements to make. No, this is no time to quit or change jobs. Job juggling won't get you pregnant anyway (remember that old myth), and you need to have a familiar schedule to fall back on when tests throw a day into chaos. But if you can lighten your job load for a month or so, it will allow you to give some attention to what's happening in your private life.

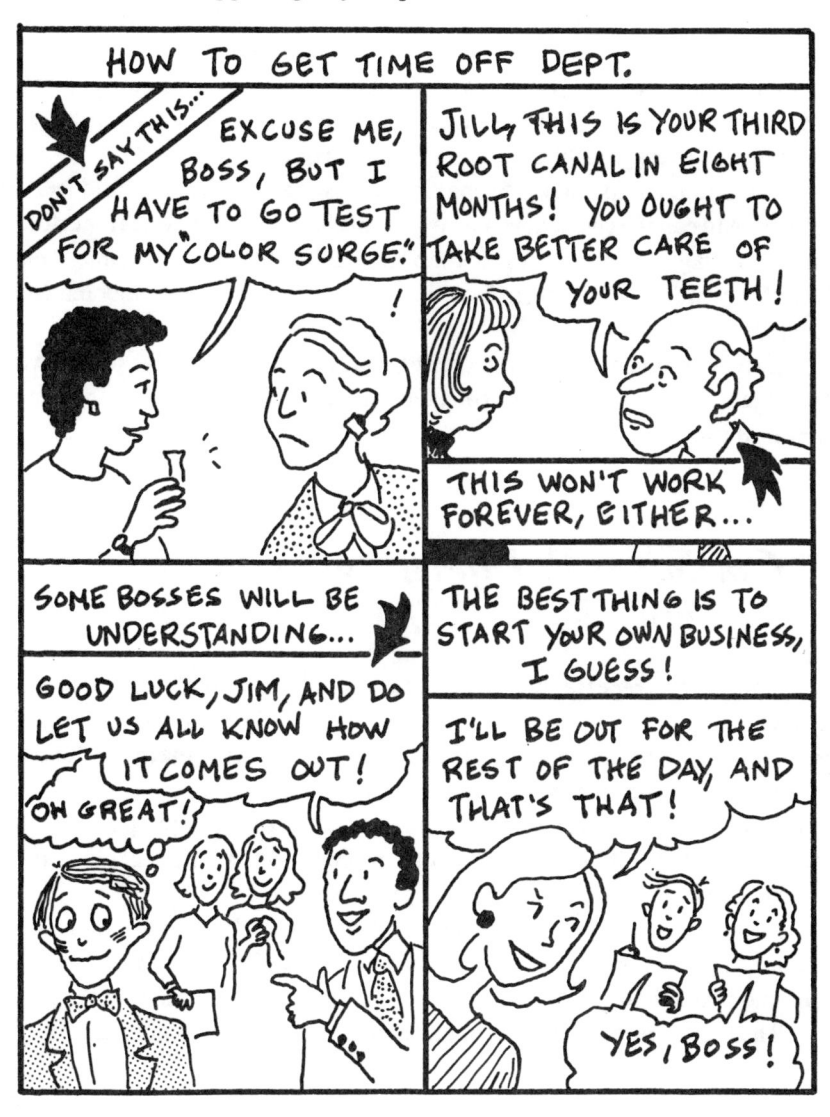

Insurance Coverage

Dealing with the bureaucracies of insurance companies is often frustrating. Add to it the job of coping with the stress of infertility testing and you have the formula for a giant headache. You are entitled to insurance coverage for workup tests, but it's up to you to see to it that you receive the coverage you deserve.

Before you begin the major workup tests, double-check your policies to make sure you understand them. Up to now, you may have used your coverage for doctors' visits and some Pap smears, so you may not fully understand how your policies function. Be prepared to become more systematic in handling your insurance paperwork so you know what reimbursements are coming to you. Go over how claims are filed for tests and office visits. Read over your hospitalization coverage, and determine if it is adequate.

Brace yourself for snafus by making copies of all claims, bills, and fees. Find out whom to call if a check goes astray. When claims are filled out at the doctor's, ask that a diagnosis more specific than "infertility" be used if possible. This will fend off potential protests from insurance carriers who may not think infertility is covered.

If treatment is ordered for either of you, you should go over your coverage once again to be sure you are protected. More discussion of insurance appears later in this book.

Coping with Infertility: Your Methods May Differ

You've read repeatedly in this book that infertility is an experience that is happening to both of you, that it is not the "fault" of one partner, that both partners should attend important medical appointments, that you should talk together about your feelings in order to cope.

What happens when the involvement level or way of coping is different for each person? What if one partner is much more upset than the other? What if one of you is resistant to infertility testing and treatment?

It can feel like the end of the world at times. You may wonder if your relationship can survive all this. You may be afraid of voicing your true feelings, thinking that keeping the peace, at least on the surface, is more important.

The first thing to realize is that although you're experiencing infertility as a couple, you remain individuals. Each of you has your own way of coping with adversity and stress in other parts of life, and chances are you are applying your methods similarly here. One of you may clam up. One of you may talk a blue streak. Sometimes a barrage of joking or crying replaces communication. Your two styles of coping may mesh together well, but often they will clash. It is unrealistic to expect yourselves to agree all the time, and it's equally unrealistic to think that you'll feel the same way about infertility all the time. This would be asking the impossible in most relationships.

This is a time when you need more support than perhaps ever before. Each of you might find yourself asking more of your partner than is possible to give right now. And ironically, this could be a time when you deeply realize, for the first time, how different you each can be. You may sometimes feel lonely, or you may feel hurt and angry.

This can also be a time when you reach a new understanding of what commitment means. You cannot demand that your partner feel exactly the same way you do. Your partner is a separate person, with separate needs. You must give your partner the right to have individual feelings. Don't blame your partner for behaving differently than you would or for worrying about the "wrong" things or not worrying about the "right" things. Recriminations just will not work.

Search for areas of compromise. Back off for a while. Try to keep talking, even if you have to change the subject a lot. Acknowledge that each of you is entitled to your own feelings, no matter what they are. Realize that there will be times when one of you will be needier than the other. At these times, try to devote special energy to your partner, even if you have to reach deeply into your emotional reserves to do it.

Coping with your differences at this time is a challenge, but it is only one of many you will face together through the years. Try to place your current situation within the perspective of your entire relationship. Move forward in time, then look back at yourselves now. You will solve this problem and move on. But, you will have learned invaluable skills about commitment along the way. You'll have learned about one another's deepest feelings; you'll see your partner in a light you'd never imagined before. Emerging from infertility, strengthened as a couple, is your goal. And, it is rewarding, indeed!

The Woman's Workup

The Physical and Pelvic Exam

You may elect to go ahead and have your initial examinations during your first office visit with your infertility specialist. Or you may make an appointment to return, giving you time to think about what you've learned during your consultation.

The very first step in any woman's infertility workup must be a general assessment of her physical condition and a pelvic examination. Your vital signs will be recorded, as in any physical. Your doctor will be checking your overall state of health, looking into your eyes, listening to your heart and lungs, and more. These ministrations will undoubtedly be familiar to you. Next, the evidence of secondary sexual characteristics will be checked. This means the doctor will look for clues that your hormones are functioning at about normal levels. These outward signs include appearance of breasts, and pubic, body, and facial hair. You'll be asked about your energy level. Are you frequently tired? Be sure to mention this to the doctor. These signs will be checked with blood testing for hormone levels, but any outward sign of a possible abnormality should be picked up now.

This part of your exam should take just a few careful minutes of observation and discussion. Next will be your pelvic exam. First the doctor will look over the general outer appearance of the genital area, looking for signs of infection, disease, or any abnormality. A speculum will be inserted into the vagina to hold its walls apart for interior examination. This does not hurt, though a metal speculum might be cold.

The doctor will visually examine the vagina and the cervix, which is the opening to the uterus. In this exam scarring, growths, signs of infection, or evidence of congenital abnormality will be sought. Also, the cervix will be checked for shape and position. Cervical mucus and the os (the cervix's opening to the uterus) will be examined, and its condition corresponding to your cycle day will be assessed.

Your specialist knows that this is the time to catch up with any vaginal diseases, chronic, common, or exotic. Do you have recurring itching or discharge? Even if you have no symptoms the day you are examined, let your doctor know. Signs of any sexually transmitted diseases may be found, and if any are suspected, cultures will be taken. You will be given a routine Pap smear if you have not had one recently.

There is a manual exam to establish the shape, position, and size of the reproductive organs. Actually it's "bimanual" in that the doctor needs both hands to feel the uterus, ovaries, and tubes. The doctor is also looking for signs of adhesions, endometriosis, scar tissue, fibroids, or any inflammation that could indicate infection. This manual exam should not be painful. It will be uncomfortable for just a few seconds. If you do feel pain, tell the doctor, for this may be a sign of an abnormality. Don't just be brave and say nothing; speaking up could help pinpoint a problem.

Is the doctor telling you what's going on as your exam progresses? If not, do a little prompting by asking, "What are you looking for now?" or a similar question. Be sure you understand what's happening if the doctor seems to have found something unusual. Anything that seems abnormal in the physical or pelvic exam will be double-checked with more sophisticated tests, so you will want to know if the physician is tracking a possible problem. Make a note of the preliminary finding now and follow along with the search.

If everything is deemed normal and healthy, be glad. You aren't out of the woods yet, but some of the physical causes of infertility have now been ruled out. But whether your doctor finds you normal or suspects a problem, you can feel good that you are now on the way to finding an answer. Often just getting through this first exam is enough to relieve lots of the anxiety that you may have felt up to now.

Tracking Your Ovulation

Interpreting Your BBT Charts During the course of your first physical and pelvic exam, your most recent charts of your basal body temperatures will be studied. If you have been keeping them, you've made a head start. If you have not, your doctor may instruct you to do so at this meeting.

If your doctor doesn't use BBT charts to help track ovulation, you should know why. The alternatives are often frequent and expensive blood testing, two or more endometrial biopsies, or repeated use of urine testing kits. BBTs are not definitively acurate, but they do give a rough picture of your cycle for far less expense and effort.

Most specialists do use at least a few months' charts to see if the sign of a temperature rise, possibly indicating ovulation, appears. As the doctor looks over your charts, you'll see what signposts are being noted. Reading these charts is somewhat subjective, so ask your doctor how yours are being interpreted. Here are some questions you may consider asking:

- Does the length of the cycle appear normal?
- Is my cycle distinctly bi-phasic (two phases)?
- Does the chart show a temperature rise?
- Does the second (or luteal) phase seem normal?
- Is there a dip in temperature before my period?
- If the chart seems abnormal, what might it mean?
- Are we keeping track of all the information you need?
- How long should we keep temperature charts?
- Do you use charts to time other tests?

Blood Work The next most simple way of tracking not only evidence of ovulation but the performance of other hormones is through blood analyses.

It is too expensive and inconvenient to run daily blood tests to track hormonal activity in your body. But your specialist will probably want to run two or three tests over the course of a cycle, at certain key times, to see what's up.

Your blood sample will be analyzed for presence of certain hormones crucial in the ovulation process. Early in your cycle, testing for the presence of FSH (follicle-stimulating hormone), LH (luteinizing hormone), progesterone, and estrogen will give a baseline for activity later in the month. Around the time of ovulation (Days 12 to 14 or so of a twenty-eight-day cycle) a blood test should be done, as well as a test near the end of the cycle, around Days 20 to 24.

These tests won't be cheap, and you may not like giving blood three times or more in one month. But the information to be gained is very valuable. Ask your doctor to go over the results with you, and explain, in simple terms, your "hormonal health." If you have a good idea about how these amazing chemicals are working in your body, you'll understand the logic behind some of the treatments that may be recommended for you.

The endometrial biopsy, which is discussed later, also confirms that ovulation has occurred by studying a snippet of the uterine lining. If the endometrium is normal and shows the proper amount of progesterone, it can be assumed that you did ovulate.

Ultrasound can be used to actually monitor the ovary and watch a follicle enlarge to release an egg. This is not usually done for simple ovulation testing, but it is commonly used to track follicle development associated with the use of fertility drugs.

The Sims-Huhner, or Postcoital, Test

What It Is, What to Expect You'll hear both of these names associated with this test. Regardless of how it is identified, this test is valuable as the first chance your doctor has to see how your partner's sperm is interacting with your cervical mucus.

Because it is the woman who must appear at the doctor's to be examined, this is often considered a "female" test, but it is important for both of you. Not only do you both participate in preparing for the test (you are instructed to make love beforehand), but clues can be found that can affect the workup plans for either one of you. Try to make this a completely shared experience by going to the doctor's office together.

The test does involve some planning and emotional commitment from each of you. Using a urine-testing kit, you'll be asked to make love as close to the time of ovulation as you can guess. Often the doctor will find it sufficient to ask you to make love the evening before a morning examination, but some doctors will want couples to make love early that same morning. Do talk over with yours what kind of time latitude you can have, and why. In many cases, making love and rushing into the office is not necessary. If this approach is favored by your doctor, it is your right to question the reason and to diplomatically mention if this scheduling is a hardship for you.

The actual examination is no more difficult than having a Pap smear. After placing a speculum in the vagina, the doctor will aspirate a sample of your cervical mucus from the opening of the cervix and from just inside the cervical canal leading toward the uterus. The samples are then evaluated for the quality of the mucus itself and for how the sperm have penetrated it and how well they can swim in it.

The mucus is checked for quantity, too—how much is being produced? If you are indeed at or close to ovulation, your cervix should be producing more mucus, and it should be clear and elastic. This elastic quality is called "spinnbarkeit," or just "spinn." A drop of the mucus will be placed between two glass slides, then the two slides will be separated to see how far the thread of mucus will stretch without breaking. The longer the stretch the better. This sounds like an odd way to look for infertility, but this stretchy, thread-like quality gives sperm a defined "lane" to swim in and promotes their trip upward into the uterus and beyond.

Some of the mucus is allowed to dry on a glass slide, then the slide is checked for a quality called "ferning." If cervical mucus dries in this fern-like pattern, it indicates the presence of adequate amounts of estrogen.

The pH of the mucus is evaluated, for the important reason that sperm cannot survive in too acid an environment. Through most of the month, the vagina is a very acidic place, but at mid-cycle the mucus should be alkaline enough to allow sperm to survive and get swimming.

After looking over the mucus, the second big job of the postcoital test begins. The mucus will be placed on a slide, under a 400-power microscope, and the sperm swimming in it will be observed. The visual field seen under the microscope is divided into sections, called high-power fields (HPF). The number of sperm counted within one of these high-power fields is a measure of how well they are surviving in your mucus. Taking into consideration how many hours have elapsed since you made love, the doctor will count live, swimming sperm, look over other sperm and debris in the sample, and form an idea of how well the sperm and mucus interact.

A count of ten live sperm per HPF is considered about the minimum, with up to about twenty-five considered very good. The motion the swimmers are making is studied, with a deliberate forward motion considered good. By the way, counting sperm during a postcoital test is not a substitute for a thorough semen analysis. Even before this postcoital test is scheduled, the man should already have had his first analysis and the results should be in the hands of the doctor at this moment. Referring to the semen analysis readings during the postcoital test gives very valuable information about the health of the sperm both in and out of your cervical mucus. If there is a possibility of an interaction problem between the two, it will be evident now.

If you hear your doctor using the term "hostile mucus," be alert. This very upsetting, almost judgmental term is used by some doctors to describe the adverse qualities of mucus that affect sperm, such as high acidity and antibody or immune reactions. Don't let this term throw you. It does not mean that you hate your partner's sperm or that your real secret wish is not to become pregnant. You may have to be treated in order to make your cervical mucus better able to support sperm, but this has nothing to do with your mental or emotional attitude.

As the doctor finishes the evaluation, ask to look under the microscope if you like. Then, be sure to have all the results explained to you so that you understand what has been discovered. If there is any area of abnormality, you will probably be asked to have another postcoital test at some point. You may need further tests for infection or immune reactions, and the man may need additional testing as well. Track the findings as your workup progresses.

NOTES

Make notes here of your discussion with your doctor about your physical and your pelvic exam:

Physical Exam

Pelvic Exam

_____
_____
_____
_____
_____
_____
_____
_____

Blood Work

Cultures or Smears Taken

_____
_____
_____
_____
_____
_____
_____
_____

NOTES

Notes on Analysis of BBT Charts

_____
_____
_____
_____
_____
_____
_____
_____
_____
_____

Blood Work for Hormones:

_____
_____
_____
_____
_____
_____
_____
_____
_____
_____

RECORD OF POSTCOITAL EXAMINATIONS

	Test One	Test Two

Date of test: _____

Time of test: _____

Time elapsed from intercourse: _____

Day of cycle: _____

Temp today: _____

Doctor performing test: _____

Mucus evaluation: _____
_____

Spinnbarkeit: _____
_____
_____

Volume: _____
_____
_____

Ferning: _____
_____

pH: _____
_____

Other notes: _____
_____
_____

Sperm per HPF: _____
_____

_____

Motility: _____

_____

_____

Overall evaluation: _____

_____

_____

What do we do next? _____

_____

_____

It's natural to be anxious about an upcoming postcoital test. Making love by the calendar is strange enough, but knowing that in a few hours the doctor will examine "how we did" can be downright stressful. Try to remind yourselves that you are indeed NOT being graded. You aren't being judged by how well you make sperm, how well you produce mucus. This is, however, an important way to find out what's happening when the two meet.

Talk together about this test before you schedule it and try to be mentally prepared for it when the proper time comes. If you can both understand how valuable its information can be to your investigation, and how absurd it can be, you will have a realistic, balanced attitude.

Your Cervical Mucus Is Gorgeous

LISA GIBLIN THELEN

a year and a half ago, my husband and I went to our infertility specialist for a postcoital test. We had set the date by looking at my temperature chart and choosing the approximate day of ovulation for the appointment. The nurse instructed me over the phone to have intercourse two to three hours beforehand, to lie flat for an hour afterward, and not to douche.

Since our appointment was for 8:15 A. M., we were supposed to have intercourse at about 5:30 that morning—something we certainly hadn't done before. After lying down for the requisite time and enjoying an extra hour of sleep, I showered and we drove to the clinic.

Although I'd been assured that the test was painless (it was), I was anxious nonetheless. As I stepped up to the examination table, I asked my doctor to explain the procedure as he went, step by step. He did, and at that point I congratulated myself on having become a more assertive patient.

After placing the speculum, the doctor used a syringe to draw out a small amount of fluid, remarking, "Your cervical mucus is gorgeous—you win the beautiful mucus award for the week." Aspirating the mucus took less than a minute. After I'd dressed, I brought my husband in from the waiting room and we both looked at the sample under the microscope. It was exciting to see the sperm swimming around, and our doctor told us that the number, shape, and motility of the sperm were all "better than excellent." We left the clinic and went out for breakfast.

Although the test result was normal, I felt sad afterwards, and my eyes kept filling up during breakfast. We are infertile because my tubes are damaged, and I thought to myself, "All those sperm with nowhere to go." I was frustrated to realize that even though I ovulated normally, had "gorgeous" cervical mucus, and was assured that my husband's sperm were healthy, I still couldn't conceive. I also felt guilty that it was me who was causing the problem. Back in college, my husband and his roommate used to fantasize about what it would be like to be fathers someday, and I felt that by marrying me, he had lost his dream of parenthood.

For me, the postcoital test aroused mixed feelings—relief that at least part of my reproductive tract was normal, frustration in still being unable to conceive, and sadness at the loss of our dream. These feelings have lessened with time, but that morning will always be a sad memory for me.

The Instructions Are Simple Enough

AMY DUECKMAN

"Well, honey, the doctor says we have to make love the morning of the sixteenth."

The instructions are simple enough: have intercourse in the morning (or possibly the night before) and come in for an examination afterwards. Sounds simple and even enjoyable at first, but is it? What if your husband works odd hours and has to leave at some ungodly hour of the morning? Do you set your alarm for 5:00 A.M. and hope you're awake enough to do what needs to be done? What if one of you, or worse, both of you, aren't in the mood? Ironically, knowing you have to do it can be the mood killer in itself. And no one tells you how you'll feel as you engage in cold, mechanical sex when your heart, mind, and body are not at all in it.

Hours later, in the doctor's office, you're asked very matter-of-factly at what time you had intercourse that morning. And you try not to be embarrassed as you answer, remembering that your doctor is really not trying to pry into your love life but is asking the question from a strictly scientific point of view. Still, you think, when else in married life, with the possible exception of your wedding night, is anyone else aware of a specific sexual encounter between you and your mate? Now, not only does the doctor know about it, but he ordered it, and he's about to reduce your lovemaking to a slide under the microscope, and examine it.

I was so relieved when later, as I explained the inconvenience of this test to my doctor, he nodded with understanding. "Sometimes all this scheduling can be a bit of a strain, can't it? Especially for the husband," he added, "because he's the one who has to get the erection." I really appreciated this caring, frank, and sympathetic attitude from my doctor. Realizing he was aware of the difficulties of these procedures helped me immensely.

Hysterosalpingogram

What It Is, What to Expect This test has the longest name of all the basic tests either of you will have. If you master the name, you will know what this test does.

- *hystero:* refers to the uterus
- *salping:* refers to the fallopian tubes
- *gram:* refers to x-rays (radiology)

This test will be ordered for you to check if your fallopian tubes are open (or "patent"). The doctor will also see on the x-rays if the inside of the uterus is normal in shape and free from obvious adhesions, scar tissue, or fibroids.

Up to this point in your workups, if no outstanding cause for infertility has been found in the blood work, temperature charts, semen analysis, or postcoital test, or if tubal problems are suspected, you should expect to have a hysterosalpingogram. It has become a very common test in an infertility evaluation. It has replaced a test that yields far less information, called the Rubin's insufflation test. This test literally blew gas into the uterus and up the fallopian tubes. A woman's painful reaction showed that her tubes were open, and that the gas had escaped into the body cavity. If a Rubin's test is suggested for your tubes, it's a sign that your doctor isn't keeping up with progress being made in infertility testing. You should consider getting another opinion, and maybe a new doctor.

The hysterosalpingogram could be scheduled before or after your endometrial biopsy. It depends on what your doctor wants to know first, or how quickly your workup is being completed. These two tests are often performed during the same cycle, and for a compelling reason: you should probably not try to get pregnant during this month. There may be a slight danger of radiation to the egg if the hysterosalpingogram is not scheduled before ovulation, and the endometrial biopsy risks losing a brand new conceptus in the womb. So, if you're having both these tests and you dislike the idea of missing too many months of trying, ask about scheduling these tests accordingly.

The hysterogram (for short) is usually performed by a radiologist, who is a physician specializing in making various x-rays. You will probably have to visit your doctor's affiliated hospital or the radiologist's office. Plan ahead for both of you to attend this test. If your partner cannot accompany you, bring a friend or relative to drive you home. Before you go to the test, ask your regular specialist about taking a very mild pain medication for cramps, such as Motrin, about an hour before your test. (If you don't have this medication on hand, you'll have time to get some.) Taking this medication is just a precaution; it doesn't mean you're bound to have terrible pain. What it does mean is that you are prepared for any possible discomfort or cramping that may occur.

For this test, you'll be asked to wear an examination or hospital gown. An assistant to the radiologist will prepare you and will ask you to lie down on a special examination table. As the radiologist prepares to begin, ask that each step of the procedure be explained to you as you go. Ask that the monitor screen be tilted so that you can turn your head slightly to see it. Both the assistant and the doctor should be happy to give you a play-by-play, and it is fascinating to see your uterus and tubes appear on a screen.

The radiologist will insert a regular speculum in the vagina and will examine your vagina and cervix carefully. Your cervix will be swabbed to prevent infection. A clamp will be placed on the side of the cervix to hold it open and in place for the test. This action will pinch and probably hurt, possibly feeling like a hefty menstrual cramp. Breathe deeply and concentrate on the procedure if you can. Listen to the radiologist as you're told about what is being discovered.

When the cervix is properly placed, a dye will be injected into the uterus, which will make the uterus and tubes appear in silhouette on the x-ray screen. There's a "live" picture on the screen, which you can watch, and the doctor will shoot stills, or x-ray films, as a record.

When the dye goes in, you'll experience some cramping and a feeling of being "full." Your body may feel like it ought to push down and expel it, but try to keep still and watch the screen. Concentrate on your breathing, and keep talking to the assistant and the doctor. The test should last no more than twenty or thirty minutes at the most. When the instruments are removed, you'll feel an immediate sense of relief, but you can expect some residual cramping. A gentle radiologist, an understanding assistant, support from your partner or a friend, and a mild pain medication go a long way toward making this test as easy on you as possible.

Immediately after the test, you'll know if your tubes are open, and you'll have a pretty good idea about the condition of your inner uterus. Getting this information so quickly is gratifying. If you haven't been given a summary of the findings, ask as you finish. Your own specialist will be studying the x-ray films and will give you an opinion also. Any questions you may have should wait until you are back with your doctor.

If signs of abnormality or infection are found, ask the radiologist before you leave if you need to take an antibiotic as a precaution. The motion of the dyes sweeping out of your tubes brings a slight chance of spreading any bacteria present, and an antibiotic is a good preventive. Call your specialist when you get home, give this information, and ask for any instructions.

Have your partner or friend drive you home. You may be feeling tired, and you'll want to rest. You may have a little spotting, which is normal. If you see more, call your specialist. If you feel at all feverish or ill, call without delay, just to be sure. Do not douche, have vaginal intercourse, or use tampons for about forty-eight hours.

Remember, the incidence of any side effects from the hysterosalpingogram is very, very low. In fact, there is one intriguing positive side effect of the hysterogram: slight obstructions inside fallopian tubes could be dislodged by the dye, thus unblocking the tube without further treatment! So, go home and take it easy—you've earned the right.

RECORD OF HYSTEROSALPINGOGRAM

Date performed: _____

Day of cycle: _____

Radiologist: _____

Results sent to Dr.: _____

_____

_____

Assessment of tubes: _____

_____

_____

Assessment of uterus: _____

_____

_____

Overall findings, as I understand them: _____

_____

_____

Side effects (if any): _____

_____

_____

Medication taken: _____

_____

_____

I've Been on Both Sides of the X-Ray Equipment

DENISE WUSINICH

*h*ysterosalpingogram—the term is long enough to scare anyone. I first heard this word when I was studying to be an x-ray technician. Little did I know I would be experiencing one firsthand. Now I've been on both sides of the x-ray equipment.

When I became a technician, "salps" were routine, always done in the afternoons. After barium enemas all morning, salps were a breeze. I used to see so many women with so many different reactions. I thought the ones who cried were being somewhat childish because some women didn't even flinch. Then I got married and left x-ray.

I tried to conceive, and after a year, I told my gynecologist. He ordered tests, which included the salp. As I entered the x-ray department for my test, I started to remember all those women to whom I'd given my hand to hold. Now it was my turn.

I had to wait an hour—my doctor had an emergency C-section (great news). When he finally came down, I was changed into a hospital gown, which looked really nice with no stockings and high heels on! The room was cold. I lay on the table, and the technician took a test film to be sure I was positioned properly. My doctor finally came in.

The first step was inserting the speculum (cold as usual!), then the uterus was clamped into position—that hurt like menstrual cramps. Dye was inserted via a long tube into the uterus. The doctor and technician watched the dye going through the uterus and coming out the tubes. I was lucky—my tubes were open and the dye spilled out. After a series of x-rays was taken, everyone but the technician left to see the films. I had pain but it wasn't too bad. After seeing that the films were correctly taken, the doctor removed the instruments and I could get dressed.

I had cramps and some bleeding. Even though I was a technician, I didn't know what the salp would be like until I experienced it. I thought it would hurt but it wasn't unbearable. Knowing it was all "for the cause" made all the difference, made it worthwhile. I went home, drank some orange juice, and slept for a few hours.

Endometrial Biopsy

What It Is, What to Expect The endometrial biopsy is a laboratory examination (biopsy) of a woman's uterine lining (endometrium) just before the onset of menstruation. Through the study of this tissue, your doctor can determine if hormones are functioning properly to develop the endometrium to nourish a fertilized egg. Progesterone plays a dominant role in the lining's formation each month, and the level of this hormone is a big part of the biopsy's findings. If an ovary has released an egg normally, the ruptured egg follicle on the ovary should be secreting progesterone. You can see that its marked presence in this test indicates that you did ovulate.

It's important to have this test during a month when you're using birth control. Or, if you like, you can have a serum pregnancy test (a lab or your doctor can take the blood sample) a day or so beforehand. The biopsy is made toward the end of your cycle, so there is a possibility of pregnancy if you have had unprotected intercourse. The doctor quickly strips away only a tiny piece of the uterine lining, so the chance of disturbing a new pregnancy is very small. Still, for peace of mind, you will want to be sure.

Watch your BBT chart as instructed by your doctor, and if you see a temperature rise, count the number of days elapsed afterward. Give this number and the day number of your cycle to the doctor the day of the test. After the test, call in to report Day 1 of your next cycle. This gives the fullest picture of the menstrual cycle in which you had your biopsy.

Find out in advance if you can take a mild pain medication, such as Motrin, an hour or so before the test. This simple precaution will help in case you have any cramping during the biopsy. You should plan to come together to the doctor's, for support and to keep the workups a shared experience.

For the test, you'll lie on the doctor's exam table, just as for a regular pelvic examination. As you begin, ask for a play-by-play as the test goes along. A speculum will first be inserted to keep the vagina open for the test. Next, the cervix will be held in place with a small clamp. Women react differently to this part of the biopsy; some feel a sensation similar to menstrual cramping, while others do have some pain. Very rapidly, the doctor will reach into the uterus with a special instrument and strip away a tiny sample of the endometrium. The instrument, called a curette, is immediately withdrawn, and the cervix unclamped. With this, you're finished.

You might have some slight spotting after the test. Expect to be instructed on douching, use of tampons, and intercourse for the first day or so after the test.

If you aren't given these details, ask. There are no side effects from this test.

The results of the endometrial biopsy won't be known for a few days or more. The tissue sample must be sent to a pathology lab for analysis. When the report comes back your doctor will go over it with you and explain what it shows. The lab should send back a "count" of how many days past ovulation your progesterone level shows. Does it approximate the number of days shown on your calendar? It should be within forty-eight hours or so. If there is a discrepancy of more than forty-eight hours, you will probably need more tests for hormone levels.

If your biopsy comes up timed properly and with a good endometrial lining, you are well on the way to clearing up worries about ovulation problems.

RECORD OF ENDOMETRIAL BIOPSY

Date of test: _____

Cycle day: _____

Date of temperature rise on BBT: _____

Next period began: _____

Doctor performing test: _____

_____

Lab's analysis: _____

_____

_____

_____

Day of cycle: _____

_____

_____

_____

Overall assessment of result: _____

_____

_____

_____

What's next? _____

_____

_____

_____

My Endometrial Biopsy

AMY DUECKMAN

I lay on the examining table and tried to get comfortable as I arranged the drape across my lower anatomy. It would be a few minutes before the doctor returned to perform the endometrial biopsy, the second test in my infertility workup, which had begun earlier that month. I didn't know what to expect, but I didn't anticipate anything pleasant.

Because the endometrial biopsy involves dilation of the cervix, I had brought along pain relievers today, just in case. "Please," I prayed silently. "Don't let it hurt too much."

It seemed to take the doctor forever to get back. I was nervous and restless to get it over with, and all there was to look at on the wall was a poster, obviously intended for mothers-to-be, telling of the importance of using car seats for children.

Presently, my doctor returned, and he proceeded with the biopsy. He inserted the speculum and then reached in with his other instrument. "Now you'll probably feel something like a menstrual cramp," he told me as he grasped the cervix, and just then, I did. It did feel like a strong cramp, and I remember being somewhat awed that this male gynecologist, who'd never experienced a menstrual cramp in his life, was telling me exactly what I should be feeling—and he was right. Fortunately, the whole procedure lasted only about half a minute. The doctor said something about having gotten a "real good sample," and I saw him drop a couple of pieces of tissue into a jar of preservative. These, he explained, would be analyzed in the lab for presence of progesterone.

I had only slight spotting afterwards and no pain. I decided it hadn't been as awful as I had prepared myself for.

Seven months later, when I underwent another biopsy, I knew what to expect. My doctor commented that I seemed to have a high pain threshold, and though I didn't say so aloud, I was thinking, "Guess I better get used to it. I figure childbirth is ten times worse."

Diagnostic Laparoscopy

What It Is, What to Expect Not every woman's workup will include this test. When your workup is in progress, as your doctor begins to put together newly discovered information from other tests, your case will be continually reevaluated, and a diagnosis will begin to emerge.

By this point the doctor:

- **will have found** nothing unusual, so a laparoscopy will be needed to provide even more information;
- **suspects the presence** of endometriosis or pelvic adhesions, which can only be confirmed by laparoscopy;
- **has found major** problems with ovulation, sperm production, or mucus, and will begin treatment. Some doctors will now put off or eliminate the laparoscopy until the success of these first treatments can be seen. Ask your doctor how definitively endometriosis or other external tubal or uterine problems can be ruled out. In cases of infertility with multiple causes, delaying a laparoscopy can sometimes mean lost time.

It's a big decision to rule out a diagnostic laparoscopy, but it's an equally big decision to have it. This test is actually a minor surgical procedure, and most are performed in the hospital under general anesthesia. It is the most expensive test to boot—involving surgeon's fees, an anesthesiologist, operating-room fees, etc. You could be staying overnight in the hospital, or you can save money by scheduling day surgery for your laparoscopy. Go over your alternatives carefully together, and talk to your doctor.

Your specialist may be a surgeon, and thus will perform the laparoscopy personally. If this isn't the case, you will be referred to a surgeon, preferably a skilled microsurgeon. Some repair work removing adhesions or endometrial implants can be done during the laparoscopy if the condition is not too severe. Ask your specialist or surgeon if there will be a videotape record made of your surgery. This will virtually eliminate the need for a second diagnostic laparoscopy should you desire a second opinion later on.

Be sure to ask if any additional procedures will be performed at the time of the laparoscopy. Sometimes the surgeon will do an additional dye study, as in a hysterosalpingogram, to check tubal patency. Often a D & C will be done to provide tissue for additional study. Ask if these extra procedures are absolutely necessary, and be sure you understand the reasons given.

As you discuss your coming laparoscopy, go over with your doctor what preoperative tests will be needed, such as chest x-rays or blood work. You should schedule these a week or so beforehand, and be sure to add these costs to the total for this test. Ask the doctor for a rundown on any side effects from any of the procedures that are being done, what bed rest will be ordered for you, any medication you might need. Ask about any lifestyle adjustments, from sexual abstinence to bathing habits, you'll have to make.

After all this advice you might be getting anxious about this procedure, but these precautions apply to any minor surgery you'd have at any time. The laparoscopy is so minor and leaves so tiny a scar that it has been dubbed the "Band-Aid" operation.

You will be told not to eat after midnight the evening before your laparoscopy. You will check into the hospital outpatient surgical unit the following day. If you're in the hospital, you check in the night before. You'll see your surgeon and your anesthesiologist beforehand, too.

As you are prepared for surgery, the anesthesiologist will give you an injection or IV to start you on a sedative. You may be asked to climb onto the operating table yourself. Once on the table, you'll be asked to count backwards, the anesthesia will kick in, and you'll fall asleep.

During this procedure, the surgeon will make a tiny incision just below the navel and will insert an instrument called a laparoscope through it. The laparoscope allows the doctor to see into your abdominal cavity to check for endometriosis, other damage, or scarring. Seeing the organs clearly is facilitated by pumping a little carbon dioxide into the abdomen first.

Using the scope, which is like a tiny telescope with a light and a fiber-optic "camera" attached, you will be examined. Evidence of recent ovulation can be checked by looking at the ovaries for signs of a ruptured follicle. Patches of endometrial tissue can be seen now, too. The condition of the fimbria, the ends of the fallopian tubes, are seen as well. Adhesions or scar tissue from past surgery, infections, or bleeding will be observed. In cases where endometriosis, scarring, or adhesions aren't very severe, repair work can be done during your laparoscopy, right then and there. Ask your surgeon in advance how this will be accomplished. If repair work is done, expect a second, small incision at the top of the pubic hairline, which will be from a second opening made for instrument use.

Once the examination, minor repairs, and additional tests are completed, the carbon dioxide will be excised from the abdominal cavity, the laparoscope withdrawn, and a few small stitches will close the incision. The average laparoscopy lasts between thirty and forty-five minutes, so you will not be under anesthesia for very long. You go to the recovery room, where you probably will wake up promptly. You'll be very groggy and maybe queasy. Your partner will come to see you, if it's allowed. Your anesthesiologist will come over to check you, and you may see your surgeon. Your memory of all this post-op business will be very hazy, so have your partner handle the talking and arrangements for you.

When you've been in recovery for a while, you'll be checked by the staff to see if you've regained your bladder function. All this means is, can you urinate without assistance? You'll go back to your hospital room (if you're checked in) or you'll get ready, slowly, to go home.

There are a few minor side effects or complications to watch out for, but for the most part, laparoscopies are performed absolutely without incident. You might feel nauseated by the anesthetic, and you'll feel groggy for some hours. You may have sharp pains in your neck and shoulder from bubbles of carbon dioxide left in the abdominal cavity. It is normal for a little of it to remain inside, and it will be absorbed by the body by the following day. If you lie down, the bubbles can't rise, hit your inside organs, and give you pain. Watch your incision and keep it clean. Any undue redness or discharge should be reported to your doctor. You may have been given some pain medication, which you will be instructed to take as needed.

You'll know results from this procedure right away. Any new lab results from the D & C will come in a few days. You'll be asked to come to the doctor's in one to two weeks to be checked, and at this time you can have a full discussion of the results and what they mean.

RECORD OF DIAGNOSTIC LAPAROSCOPY

Date performed: _____

Hospital: _____

Surgeon: _____

Outpatient? _____

Day of cycle: _____

Findings: _____

Endometriosis found? _____

Notes: _____

Condition of ovaries: _____

Condition of tubes: _____

Any removal of adhesions or endometriosis performed? _____

Overall assessment of reproductive organs: _____

D & C performed? _____

Result: _____

Dye study? _____

Result: _____

Video record made? _____

Record held by: _____

Reaction to general anesthesia: _____

What's next? _____

A Laparoscopy Experience

KASSIE SCHWAN

*I*t is all over. I was neither a screaming baby about it, nor was I as brave as Joan of Arc, but at least it is all over.

Last Wednesday I really had a case of nerves over this laparoscopy. I had so little information on what it was really going to be like, and forging into the unknown isn't one of my favorite pastimes. I read and re-read the piddling amout of information on laparoscopy in the two infertility paperbacks that I have, but found little comfort or knowledge, since the authors, men, and the authorities cited, all male physicians, have no personal experience with this procedure! Then I pawed over the information ditto I mailed away for from RESOLVE, which gave more information than anything else, including possible complications of the surgery. That had me jumping out of my skin! Infection at the incision, embolisms into the bloodstream, internal injury to organs by an accidental swipe of the laparoscope. Goodness! Plus, I mulled over the advice of my GP, who advised to never undergo general anesthesia unless it is extremely important. Of course, how could I forget my ballet teacher's wonderful story of the man she knew who checked into the hospital for "elective" surgery and never came out again??!!

Thursday night, the night before, was very restless for me. I knew I had o'get up at 5:30, so I barely slept, and was awake by five. The sun was just coming up when my husband Brian and I left the apartment. I gave my wedding ring to him to keep, since I couldn't wear it into surgery. I made sure Brian had my list of things to ask the doctors, since I would be too groggy to do any asking anyway.

The Day Surgery Unit at the hospital wasn't even open yet, we got there so early! Brian and I sat on a couch in the hall, said good morning to the security guard, and nervously watched the early-morning traffic out the window.

The nurse finally came to get me. I changed into hospital gown and robe, and paper booties. I couldn't bring myself to put on the shower-cap-type hair covering yet. The nurse took my temperature and noticed that I had a case of the sniffles. I honestly didn't think that this slight cold could affect anything, but she was sternly concerned. "You see, your infection could be spread throughout your system by the anesthetic." She called Brian in to see me and left.

Well, now was the time for terror! If they cancelled the surgery due to the cold, I would have to go through all the agony over again, and if I did have it today, I'd be ill or dying in a matter of hours!

The anesthesiologist came in presently, and said the only complication might be that my tickly throat might be irritated by the tube he would be putting down it. He was very cool, friendly, unperturbed, and reassuring. Brian asked all the fearful questions instilled in us by the nurse, and he assured us that my minor cold would not be a factor.

Then it was really time to go. The nurse had me remove my glasses and had Brian take them. I gave him a kiss, and the nurse led me out of the cubicle and down the hall to the day surgery OR.

As I walked in, I saw my doctor, who was also cheerful and reassuring. I lay down on the table, and several professionals of various types started working on me at once! Everybody was very busy, friendly, and efficient. I guess I sounded a note of pessimism when I said to my doctor, "I hope you find something. I have waited two years to find out what's wrong." He replied, "There are things we can do. It is not hopeless." I really found solace in those words.

He left to scrub, and the anesthesiologist said, "Think of something very pleasant you want to dream about." I thought of the swimming pool at Jones Beach, and as I did so, I could feel the sleeping potion beginning to take effect. It was as if a giant, silent weight was being slowly but firmly pressed onto my body, and I was powerless to resist or fight it. It gave new meaning to the word "overwhelming." As I realized that I was about to pass out and be cut up at last, the anesthesiologist leaned over to me and said, "Can I have a little smile before you go?" With the greatest effort I managed to twitch the corners of my mouth. And then, as the romances say, I knew no more.

Coming to was an interesting experience. My brain switched on alertly enough for me to begin thinking, "This is me waking up . . . where have I been? . . . oh yes, I must be waking up from the operation . . . the nurses are mumbling something . . . I have no worries nor any knowledge of my life right now! . . . nothing . . . but it is coming back , . I am coming back . . . I am starting to remember . . . "

I first remember two nurses putting a pillow under my very heavy head. I was incredibly groggy, but I wasn't feeling the nausea that I had been warned about, and I didn't seem to have any cramping. I was truly in limbo! The anesthesiologist came over to see me several times while I was recovering, and I was grateful he was as interested in how I was waking up as how I had gone to sleep.

Brian came in about 45 minutes after I hit the recovery room, and started speaking to me in a very matter-of-fact manner. Although I could hear and understand him, I knew I just couldn't grasp the information he was telling me. I just kept repeating over and over again, "I'm so groggy!" I repeatedly reported to the anesthesiologist, "I'm so out of it!" And I kept telling the nurses, "I'm so thirsty!"

I knew I was all right, but there was great difficulty in regaining my faculties. I knew I had to become alert, that was now my job. And I felt as though it was impossible to do. It took me a long time to even be able to handle being conscious there on the bed, and I was fearful because the nurses began coming over and telling me that before long they were going to sit me up. I couldn't imagine being able to sit up! I felt as though I were trying to push my way through the thickest jungle possible. It really was a struggle.

I heard a woman on the other side of the curtain complain that she was feeling nauseated, and I thought, "Please don't say that—the power of suggestion may make me nauseated too!" When she also complained that the IV in her hand was hurting her, I became aware that I too was sporting one, but mine didn't hurt.

Brian popped in and out several times. But my doctor, the infertility specialist who did my laparoscopy, never came over to see or speak to me. I could hear his voice in the recovery room, but I didn't have the strength to call him over. I felt badly that he didn't come over . . . or maybe he did, and I don't remember?

The nurses suddenly sat me up, and that was a jolt! It took all my powers to get used to the position, and it made me dread what was coming next . . . they would get me out of bed and put me in a chair! My recovery, thus, was fraught with achievement anxiety . . . can I make it to the next stage like a good patient???

Before I knew it, the nurse had me up and slowly walking across the room. I was inside it before I realized she had walked me to the bathroom . . . "Let's see, how does one go to the bathroom . . . do I remember?" I thought to myself. She hung the IV on a hook on the door and said, "I'm right outside."

That was reassuring. I was feeling pretty helpless about then.

Concentrating on the process of the operation and the recovery helped me to blot out the reason why I was there. I did manage to hear and understand Brian telling me that they had found no endometriosis, and that I seemed perfectly healthy. He said that my doctor told him there were still things we could do, and that it was not hopeless. I knew in recovery, then, that I was healthy. I really did not want to discover I had some awful pregnancy-preventing condition, but to do all this for nothing! It was a strange feeling.

The nurses got me into the dreaded chair. Shortly thereafter, it was time for me to dress myself, get my parting instructions, and go. Brian drove slowly and tried to avoid the potholes in the streets, but the biggest obstacle was the four flights of stairs to our apartment! I went up the entire way in one burst of determination and was most proud of my tremendous achievement. I lowered myself into bed, and then . . . I had the pain that the nurses had warned me about. The carbon dioxide pumped into the abdomen during the laparoscopy, then expressed out again, doesn't all come back out. Some remains in the body cavity, and when one stands, the bubbles rise and hit the diaphragm. The nerves reacting to this cause pains in the upper chest and shoulders. And boy, does that hurt! I had so many stabbing, jabbing pains in my chest, neck, and shoulder that I was writhing and moaning, "What am I going to do??" and scaring the pants off Brian. In about ten minutes it began to recede, and I calmed down.

Now, here I am, four days later, and I've been up and about. I'm not exactly energetic, and my right shoulder still has some pain in it. I get tired really fast. My little belly-button incision has been exposed . . . I pulled off the Band-Aid. I never got the abdominal cramping they warned about, so I'm glad of that. My discharge is slight.

I'm glad that's over.

Other Tests for Women

As your infertility specialist runs through the workup tests, sometimes further investigation is needed to refine a diagnosis or to continue to seek out a yet-unfound cause of infertility.

Hysteroscopy The hysteroscopy is a cousin of the laparoscopy. If for some reason your doctor feels your uterus should be examined visually from within, a hysteroscopy will be suggested. It may be done simultaneously with a laparoscopy or it might be a separate procedure. If your doctor thinks you need a hysteroscopy, it could be scheduled as an outpatient procedure, but if a laparoscopy is also in the plans, you can probably have them performed at the same time. In doing so, you'll be subjected to anesthesia only once instead of twice.

The hysteroscope, like a laparoscope, is a tube-like device with optics that can allow the surgeon to look inside the uterus. It is usually introduced into the uterus through the cervix, so no incision is needed. If adhesions or structural problems exist, they will be discovered or confirmed now. Some minor repairs can be performed during this visual examination, too.

A scalpel-like attachment to the hysteroscope can allow some tissue to be snipped away. Lasers can also be used to vaporize adhesions during hysteroscopy. Sometimes the walls of the uterus will be kept from sticking together by the introduction of a balloon-like device that is inflated to help the uterus keep its form. You can see that many hysteroscopies are far more than diagnostic procedures alone—you may awaken from your anesthesia and find that you're all set to start trying again with new, and better, odds.

Be sure you understand why you need a hysteroscopy and what repairs will be performed during the procedure. If adhesions are suspected, see if a laser can be used rather than the traditional lysis (cutting) methods, because often less blood and scarring may result. If you have not had a hysterosalpingogram before you're scheduled for a hysteroscopy, find out why.

Radiology Work If you've had a laparoscopy or other surgery, you've had chest x-rays taken in conjunction with your workup. The experience was painless and relatively simple and probably wasn't new to you. Hysterosalpingograms, too, are radiology work. To pinpoint other diagnoses, radiology also plays a role.

If your doctor has discovered through blood tests that you have elevated levels of the hormone prolactin, you may be told that a CAT-scan is needed to discover the source. Sometimes elevated prolactin is caused by a microscopically small, noncancerous tumor of the pituitary gland at the base of the brain. They are very common and usually not serious. A CAT-scan (computerized axial tomography) takes pictures of the skull and will reveal if you have a tumor of this type.

Don't let this situation frighten you. Pin your doctor down and really talk about what is suspected, if it is a cause for concern, and how it might be treated. Often a medication taken by mouth called bromocriptine is all that's needed to control this type of tumor, so do not panic. Pituitary tumors may be common knowledge to your doctor, but they aren't to you, so don't allow this possibility to be shrugged off. Get all your questions out of the way promptly, and ask for a separate consultation to reassure yourself.

A CAT-scan is absolutely painless and noninvasive. That is, not a thing actually goes into your head. The scan is usually performed in the radiology unit of a hospital. You will lie on a table that slides through a large donut-shaped structure attached to one end. There is no pain, and there is nothing complicated for you to do during this test except to hold very still. The results will be available to your own doctor right away. The radiologist may or may not choose to discuss your results with you, so wait for the full story from your specialist. Find out if you can hold the films for safekeeping or in case you need a second opinion.

Ultrasound Ultrasound is an old friend to women taking fertility drugs, but sometimes ultrasound is used during a workup, too. Ultrasound can be used to look at the ovaries, tubes, or to search out fibroids.

Ultrasound sends out soundwaves that bounce off the internal organs in the abdomen. The echoes of this action are transformed into images that can be seen on a screen, forming a picture of what's inside. It may take some practice for you to recognize what's what on screen, but your doctor can read the shadowy images with no problem.

Traditional ultrasound is certainly painless, but requires the discomfort of a bladder that is full to bursting. The sound waves are better conducted and give a better image through water. Downing glass after glass of water and waiting for your ultrasound can be nerve-wracking as you wonder if you're going to be able to "hold it" until your test is over.

You'll probably be asked to change into an examination gown. For ultrasound you simply lie on your back on the examination table, next to the ultrasound equipment. The doctor or assistant will squeeze some clear gel onto your abdomen—this helps to conduct the sound waves.

A small, box-like instrument, called a transducer, is used to send the ultrasound signal and pick it back up after it has bounced off the internal abdominal organs. It is placed on your abdomen and drawn across it with slight pressure, until it is in the correct position. In most cases, the patient can see the image on the monitor, and can talk about it with the doctor during the procedure.

Ask your specialist about the ultrasound method that uses a vaginal transducer to send and pick up the waves. This ultrasound wand visualizes the internal organs from a vantage point already inside the body—in the vagina. This eliminates the need for the waves to travel through the outer skin. The ovaries and tubes can be better seen, and you don't need to drink bucketfuls of water.

Karyotyping   In cases of repeated miscarriages where a genetic defect is suspected, this blood test may be called for. In this test, both yours and your partner's blood will be drawn, and the chromosomal breakdown of each will be mapped out. This test is very expensive, and it takes time for the results to come back.

If a karyotype has been suggested to you, it should be in conjunction with genetic counseling. You should talk to a professional specializing in genetics who is qualified to help you grasp the implications of your tests and help you decide what you should do next. Be sure to ask if this help will be available to you.

The Man's Workup

Semen Analysis

What It Is, What to Expect   It cannot be emphasized strongly enough: a careful and comprehensive semen analysis, repeated at least twice to insure accuracy, is the absolute foundation of the man's infertility workup.

Be sure you are using a lab experienced in doing detailed semen analyses. This test constitutes far more than just counting the number of sperm cells under a microscope, and ordinary labs that don't specialize in this work may fall short of a thorough job. Ask your specialist to recommend a lab, or call your local RESOLVE and obtain a referral.

You will need two or three of these analyses to form a good picture of what's happening with sperm production and seminal fluid. It takes about ninety days for sperm to complete the manufacturing process within the man's body, so you can surmise that you will have to wait at least three months before you can double-check all you need to know. If you get started with the first analysis at the outset of both workups, the three-month interval is not an unreasonable delay, even for the most impatient.

The first analysis should take place before the postcoital test is scheduled. The second can be scheduled according to your specialist's direction, but if nothing abnormal has appeared already, having the test within five weeks or so is probably fine. If you had a cold, fever, or other infection, you may have to wait the three months to see if your earlier result was affected. If two tests are within the normal range and appear reasonably consistent, you may not need a third right away. But if the workups or treatments begin to stretch out over a longer period of time, count on having another analysis in the future, just to keep tabs on your status. Some doctors recommend this test be done every six months throughout the period when the couple is trying to conceive.

To get the most accurate picture of your normal sperm production, discuss with your doctor how long you should abstain from sex prior to producing the semen specimen. The time period ought to be comparable to your usual interval between emissions, but everybody's different. It might embarrass you to discuss something as personal as frequency of sexual relations or masturbation, but if your doctor has thoroughly taken your medical history, this topic has been raised already. If talking about this really turns you off, tell yourself that the doctor has heard it all before—nothing you say is going to be new, strange, or bad. You aren't being judged! Try to remember these things when you begin to feel uncomfortable.

The semen analysis is similar to the postcoital test, in that the man must muster up some sexual feelings in order to produce the sample that's going to be examined. With the postcoital test, you can cope together at home, but many semen samples have to be produced at the lab, which is no fun. If you can, have the doctor or the lab provide sample jars for you to use at home, and bring your specimen to the lab as quickly as possible. Unfortunately, "giving at the office" produces fresher samples which can be tested right away, and many labs prefer them.

The semen specimen is most commonly produced by means of masturbation. If your doctor or the lab gives you the choice of producing the specimen at home you may prefer to work together to bring the man to orgasm (being ready, of course, to quickly collect the ejaculated semen). It's purely a matter of personal choice. Do what makes you most comfortable. If you prefer complete privacy, explain this simply to your partner.

If you find you must produce a specimen at the lab, you won't have the choice of being together. You will be sent to a private bathroom and will be left alone for as long as you need. Some labs even provide stimulating "reading" material, but some don't. This may be shocking or funny to you but nevertheless, some men do use magazines like *Playboy* to help them get into the mood for performing in such an impersonal atmosphere. Come prepared if your lab doesn't have any, but do your partner a favor and pitch it when you leave!

Providing semen samples can be embarrassing, but once you've been through it for the first time, you're over the biggest hurdle. Subsequent semen analyses won't be a picnic, of course, but the strangeness and absurdity of this situation will begin to blot out your negative feelings. Someday you might even get to the point that you can laugh about it together—many couples do.

Ideally, the specimen should be collected into a clean, dry, wide-mouthed glass jar. The jars you get at the doctor's or lab are often plastic, and some experts feel that plastic can affect the liquefaction of the semen, but what can we do? That may be what you have to work with, and good labs will take this into account. Pick up several jars at the same time, and keep spares at home for future use. If you use a jar from home, a small peanut butter jar or something similar would do pretty well. Thoroughly wash and rinse the jar to remove any detergent residue.

Label the jar with your name, address, phone, and the date and time the sample was collected. Put in parenthesis the number of days' abstinence if your doctor or lab requires it. (Remember to make a note of it at home even if you aren't asked to provide this information.) If this labeling business embarrasses you, you can tape a blank piece of paper over the label, which can be removed by the lab worker. Stash the jar in a bag or briefcase, and no one will notice.

Be sure to deliver the specimen to the lab well within two hours. One hour is much preferable. This may be inconvenient, but it is essential to obtain the most accurate results. If getting to the lab from home takes too long, you'll probably have to consider collecting the sample at the lab instead of at home.

Some men have religious beliefs that prohibit masturbation for any reason. You may be able to have normal intercourse which you then deliberately interrupt in order to withdraw and collect your semen. (This is difficult but not impossible.) Or, your doctor can provide you with a condom-like sheath for the penis, that you can use to collect semen during completed intercourse. If you are restricted about using birth control, which the sheath collection method resembles, placing a pinhole in the sheath near the top can technically render it incomplete protection. If you can, talk to an understanding religious authority and ask for advice. RESOLVE members can help you with this problem, too.

Once the specimen gets to the lab worker, it is analyzed for a variety of important factors. Counting sperm cells alone just doesn't do the job. Looking at the sperm for shape, size, swimming ability, and maturity is just as important. The seminal fluid in which the sperm swim is examined, too. Here's a rundown on how to understand your semen analysis as it might be done step-by-step:

1. **Liquefaction**
   When seminal fluid is first produced it is in liquid form, but within a few minutes its consistency usually begins to change. It becomes gel-like for a period of about twenty or thirty minutes, then reliquefies. After it reliquefies, the lab worker measures its volume and begins the analysis. Liquefaction is best noted if the specimen is produced on the premises.

2. **Volume**
   How much seminal fluid was produced? Too little fluid will result in the sperm having a tough time swimming to the cervical mucus. Too much fluid will "water down" the sample so there are fewer sperm per measured volume of liquid. Between about two and five cubic centimeters is considered a normal range.

3. **Viscosity**
   This refers to the consistency of the seminal fluid once liquefaction has occurred. Can the sperm swim freely in a flowing liquid or are they trapped in a thicker fluid? Viscosity is measured on a scale of 0 to 4, with 0 the normal reading. This factor by itself is not crucial unless sperm motility is reduced.

4. **Motility**
   How well do the sperm swim? Swimming direction and speed are factors of good sperm motility. The analysis will give you a percentage of the sperm that are satisfactorily motile; that is, the fraction of the sperm count that are swimming forward at average to good speed. Obviously, the higher the percentage you have the better, but readings of about 60 percent are considered normal. Speed is expressed on a scale of 0 to 4, with 4 being excellent speed with good forward direction. An average of 60 percent motility analysis would comprise sperm swimming at a speed level of 2 to 3 after two hours or so.

5. **Morphology**
   Attention is also given to the shape of the sperm, or morphology.

Morphology is important because we know that only normally shaped sperm are able to fertilize an egg. Morphology is espressed as a percentage of the sperm total that is normal in shape. What's normal? An oval head, and a tapering, whipping tail. There are all kinds of abnormal shapes in any semen specimen, such as two-headed sperm, those with two tails, no tails, round or elongated heads, etc. Immature sperm cells are also found.

For conception odds to be normal to good, about 60 percent or better of the sperm examined for morphology should be normal. Poor morphology could result from an infection or from exposure to heat, so a second semen analysis should be done before morphology is confirmed as abnormal. Plus, immature sperm cells are sometimes confused with white blood cells in the ejaculate, another good reason to use a competent lab.

6. Sperm Count

At last. This is the best-known of the checks on the semen specimen—just how many sperm were produced?

Count is expressed by the number (usually in millions) per cubic centimeter (or milliliter) of volume. A representative volume of the total sample is placed in a "counting chamber" where the number observed can be extrapolated to represent the number in the entire specimen.

A count of about sixty million and above is considered good. Counts of forty million and up are considered fine if a good percentage of them is healthy and vigorous. Counts below twenty million are known as "oligospermic" and are to be carefully analyzed, though there are many pregnancies resulting from counts at this level. Pregnancy is unlikely (but not unheard of) if the count is below 10 million. Complete absence of sperm is known as "azoospermia."

Working with the sperm count alone will not give you the true picture of your semen analysis. Don't be alarmed at a low figure until you hear all the details and find out how you can be treated. Conversely, don't rest on your laurels with only one high count. You must have more than one semen analysis, no matter what the results.

7. Agglutination

If the sperm seem to be clumping together abnormally, this will be noted in the report. Sperm that bunch together cannot swim normally, and are probably clumping as a reaction to attack by antibodies present in the seminal fluid. Antibodies are agents produced by the body to eliminate foreign invaders such as germs, virus, and infection. There is some debate over how important an infertility factor sperm antibodies really are, because many men have at least some antibodies in their semen. Ask your doctor's views of this cause of infertility. If the only abnormal factor in your analysis is clumping, then it must be determined if this could really be the only reason for infertility. Don't suspend the woman's workup just because this factor has turned up. More investigation is needed.

8. **Azoospermia** (complete absence of sperm)
If no sperm are found in the seminal fluid, the reason will be sought. The first test to discover why will measure the fluid for fructose. The presence of fructose indicates a blockage that is preventing the sperm from getting through the ducts to be mixed with seminal fluid. Further tests (see the following) will be ordered.

If your first analysis comes back with normal readings, you have reason to be glad. But be sure to confirm the result with another analysis at an interval recommended by your doctor. If you have some abnormal factors, don't be discouraged. A second test is absolutely necessary to confirm any result, and some causes are indeed temporary.

You may wonder if you really need to know all this. The answer is "yes," because interpretation of the total semen analysis is somewhat subjective. To produce a pregnancy, certain factors can be enhanced by treatment of the female or of the male. Two specialists may have different opinions as to what to do. You will want a thorough explanation from your doctor as to how your analysis is read and what conclusions can be drawn. If you have a good lab, all these factors will be tested. If not, you will know to switch labs. Stay on top of your own case, because all other tests you will have will be based on what your semen analyses tell you and your doctor.

RECORD OF SEMEN ANALYSES

Under care of Dr.: _____

Lab: _____

Date of analysis: _____

Date of abstinence: _____

Volume: _____

Viscosity: _____

Agglutination: _____

Count total: _____

Count per milliliter: _____

Remarks: _____

Morphology: _____

% Normal: _____

Types of abnormals seen: _____

Remarks: _____

Motility: _____

% Motile: _____

Grade motility: _____

Remarks: _____

Overall assessment of the results: _____

Next analysis should be when? _____

RECORD OF SEMEN ANALYSES

Under care of Dr.: _____

Lab: _____

Date of analysis: _____

Date of abstinence: _____

Volume: _____

Viscosity: _____

Agglutination: _____

Count total: _____

Count per milliliter: _____

Remarks: _____

Morphology: _____

% Normal: _____

Types of abnormals seen: _____

Remarks: _____

Motility: _____

% Motile: _____

Grade motility: _____

Remarks: _____

Overall assessment of the results: _____
_____
_____

Next analysis should be when? _____

RECORD OF SEMEN ANALYSES

Under care of Dr.: _____

Lab: _____

Date of analysis: _____

Date of abstinence: _____

_____

Volume: _____

Viscosity: _____

Agglutination: _____

Count total: _____

Count per milliliter: _____

Remarks: _____

Morphology: _____

% Normal: _____

Types of abnormals seen: _____

Remarks: _____

Motility: _____

% Motile: _____

Grade motility: _____

Remarks: _____

_____

Overall assessment of the results: _____

_____

_____

Next analysis should be when? _____

I Gave at the Office

JEFFREY HUDSON

*S*ome people may think providing a sperm specimen at a doctor's office is no different than having your blood drawn. They may even think it's better. After all, there are no needles. Coming up with a sperm specimen may even sound like fun—after all, masturbation is supposed to be a pleasurable activity. Take it from me, I'd rather have someone poking a needle into my arm any day.

On a typical visit to a typical sperm laboratory, the waiting room is the first tip-off that this may not be the easiest way to spend half an hour. Usually, the room is filled with anxious men, eager to avoid any eye contact with one another. Sometimes there are couples, who converse in hushed phrases. The anonymity of a usual doctor's office is nowhere to be found. Every man knows why the others are here.

Every few minutes, a woman arrives, carrying a paper bag. It's not her lunch. While she may be embarrassed about disclosing its contents, the receptionist has no such qualms. The woman is ordered to take the small plastic bottle out of the bag and place it on the desk, and we are all presented with a full view of her partner's "contribution."

After about fifteen minutes the receptionist calls my name. I approach her desk and am told to fill out a medical information form, which asks how long it's been since my last "emission." I'd been told to wait forty-eight hours, and luckily nothing intervened to spoil the test.

I hand the form back, and then write out a check in advance. I'm told to follow a young nurse, who leads me down a series of corridors to an examination room. Handing me a sterile specimen bottle, she then sheepishly explains the "special features" of this room. Instead of medical supplies, the drawers underneath the examination table are filled with a large library of *Playboy* magazines, which I am free to "use as I see fit."

Feeling that I ought to separate myself from men who might be attracted by such material, I say that the magazines won't be necessary. The nurse makes a remark about what a great job she has, and quickly closes the door.

I look around the room, half-blinded by the bright fluorescent lighting. I hold up the specimen bottle, trying to figure out why it's made of plastic when I'm sure I read somewhere that clean glass is better. I glance at the pile of tattered magazines, and see that several of them are over five years old. How many other men have been here before me, feeling as far from desire as it's possible to feel, yet knowing that their solitary vice must now carry a larger purpose?

Several long minutes later, the task is done, though not without some difficulty and awkwardness. The bottle now contains a specimen. But things aren't over yet. I carry my "donation" down the hall to the receptionist's desk. where I must hand it to her in front of everybody else. She holds it up, writes my name on the label, and tells me I'll have the results tomorrow.

Thanking her (I don't know for what) I try to assemble what's left of my dignity, skirt past the stares I'm sure are directed at me in the waiting room, and briskly leave the office. I call my wife and tell her to pick up some specimen jars at her doctor's and keep them at home!

The Physical Exam

What It Is, What to Expect   If one or more areas of abnormality show up in your semen analysis, you will probably be referred to a urologist or andrologist specializing in male infertility problems. If you have not been referred and it looks like you may need further tests and treatment, consider finding a male infertility specialist yourself. It is as important for men as for women to find the best care possible, and most doctors who treat women do not also specialize in this area.

At your urologist's, you will give your medical history again, and you will have a physical exam. You may be asked to undergo a thorough physical with your internist, too. Signs of general health will be checked, such as blood pressure, temperature, heartbeat, etc. You will have a urinalysis, and blood may be drawn to monitor health and to get a blood count.

The urologist will look you over for outward signs of any possible hormonal imbalance, such as the pattern of hair distribution on the face and body. After this once-over, your genitals will be examined.

The penis will be checked for shape, curvature, and placement of the urethral meatus (the opening in the end of the penis). Testicle size will be measured. The doctor will gently examine the scrotum by touch. Each testicle will be checked, and the epididymis and spermatic cords (the lines which transport sperm, and the accompanying blood vessels) will also be examined manually for any abnormality. Inserting a gloved finger into the rectum facilitates an examination of the prostate gland and checks for an abnormality in the rectum itself. For this examination, you will be asked to lean over onto the examination table. It is a bit uncomfortable for a moment, but it's not painful. If there is extreme sensitivity or pain, an infection of the prostate could be the cause.

The veins running through the scrotum are examined with a simple maneuver. After standing for a few moments, you'll be asked to bear down with your muscles, as if for a bowel movement. This fills the scrotal veins with blood and makes a condition called varicocele become more apparent to the eye and to the touch.

Varicocele, or a varicose vein in the scrotum, is fairly common. The varicose vein causes blood to pool in the lower area of the scrotum, raising its temperature and hampering sperm production. Bear in mind that doctors have found varicoceles in men who have successfully fathered children, but statistically speaking, a much higher percentage of men with fertility problems have a varicocele present.

Double-checking the varicocele is done in two ways. A special stethoscope is used to listen to the blood movement in the scrotum. Plus, a thermal plate can be used to give a photographic image of the temperature variation over the entire scrotum. You'll be asked to press the scrotum against the thermal plate to give the image. The varicocele will look "hot."

This physical exam will be followed up by a discussion of the findings and their implications. You and your partner should both be present. Recommendation of further testing or treatment should be covered at this time. Double-check with the woman's specialist to be sure both doctors have all the findings. You may want to discuss your course of action with her doctor and adjust your tests and treatment planning accordingly. Be sure that you two are talking to each doctor and that the doctors have talked to one another as well.

Other Tests for the Male Workup

Blood Work If your sperm count has shown some abnormalities and you've had a physical exam, you may be asked to have some blood work done to check your hormonal levels. If your doctor wants simply to test for thyroid problems, then stimulate your thyroid gland, beware. Consider getting another opinion from an andrologist. At the very least, ask for a complete hormonal assay that includes readings of FSH, LH and testosterone. Through these tests a good lab and a specialist with an understanding of male fertility can close in on what may be causing hormonal problems.

More Tests on Semen and Sperm More sophisticated testing can be done on the semen specimen to track suspected problems. They include:

- If no sperm is found, a fructose test is automatically done by competent labs. This will confirm if there is blockage in the ejaculatory ducts.
- If there is a great deal of clumping of the sperm, tests will be run to see why the sperm are behaving this way. Infections such as ureaplasma (also called mycoplasma) are found by culturing some of the seminal fluid. You will also be asked for a urine specimen, which will be cultured as well. Chlamydia, another infection, is sought this way also. If you are being tested for these infections, be sure your spouse is tested as well. Both of these

infections are sexually transmitted, and you both will have to be treated, probably with antibiotics.

Clumping is also caused by antibodies produced by the man against his own sperm. His body, for some reason, has identified his sperm as foreign, and is trying to eliminate them. (This antibody reaction can be found in the woman, too, which often shows up in the postcoital examination.) To confirm this, your sperm will be "washed," or separated from its seminal fluid and resuspended in another liquid. If the sperm do not clump, your own seminal fluid could be causing the antibody reaction. If a poor postcoital test points to antibody problems, the woman's mucus is tested with your sperm, then a donor woman's mucus is tested with your sperm. There may only be clumping with your partner's mucus.

A hamster test might be ordered to see if your sperm can penetrate the outer skin of an egg to fertilize it. A hamster's egg has qualities similar to human ova and is used for this test. Your sperm is washed and placed in a dish with hamster ova, and if it can break through the egg's chemical skin (NO fertilization of any sort takes place), it can be assumed that it can do the same for a human egg. This test is very expensive, and you should ask exactly why it is necessary.

A "Penetrak" test checks how well the sperm swim in mucus other than that of your partner. The Penetrak is a thin glass tube filled with the mucus of an ovulating cow. Bovine mucus is quite similar to human mucus and makes a good substitute for the purposes of this test. The sperm are introduced into the tube, and how well and how quickly they swim upward is measured. This motility is measured against motility in your partner's mucus.

Invasive Tests on the Male The testicular biopsy and the vasogram are tests that are performed only when all other options and tests are played out or there is a suspicion of a specific problem. These tests, if not performed by very skillful hands, can sometimes damage delicate tissues. Be sure to discuss exhaustively the reasons why your specialist wants you to have these tests, and come to an understanding of the balance between the benefits to be realized and the small risk of damage. Consider obtaining another opinion.

If your sperm count is very low and hormone therapy is not working well enough, your doctor may want a close look at the inner workings of the testicles. This is accomplished through a testicular biopsy. The biopsy is performed in the hospital, under general anesthesia. A small wedge of tissue will be carefully excised from the testicle and studied for the presence of various cells essential to

YOUR INFERTILITY IS INVESTIGATED: THE WORKUPS 113

the process of sperm production. The biopsy can show if an obstruction is causing the problem, if there is an absence of sperm-manufacturing cells, or if there is an arrest in the process of sperm maturation. Be sure you understand what your specialist is looking for, why, and what treatments might be recommended as a result of the findings. In the biopsy, a small incision is made on the scrotum, then a wedge of tissue is obtained from the testicle. It is a simple procedure, but very exacting and delicate. You can probably have this done on an outpatient basis, so ask.

The pain resulting from this procedure should not be severe, but there will be some swelling of the scrotum. Ice packs placed against the scrotum can help. The incision should heal quickly, and any pain should disappear in one to two days. Monitor your own recovery and call your doctor should anything seem amiss.

A vasogram is an x-ray of the sperm ducts and is usually used to pinpoint a suspected blockage. The image showing the blockage location is the road map used by the doctor if you are having surgery to correct the blockage. Sometimes a vasogram is performed before a testicular biopsy. Whether it's done as a part of other surgery or not, it is always done under general anesthesia. The duct known as the vas deferens is injected with opaque dye that fills the ducts, epididymis, and other tissues. These then show up on the x-rays.

Be sure you need these two tests. Any surgery requiring general anesthesia is not to be taken lightly, and these tests aren't just to satisfy general curiosity. There ought to be plenty of prior evidence to justify the biopsy and the vasogram. Finding a skillful doctor to perform these tests is a good idea. Ask for a referral, get another opinion, or call on RESOLVE for some names.

SECTION III
Your Infertility Treatment

*t*reatment will begin once your doctor has diagnosed an infertility problem. You might be given medication or be advised that corrective surgery or procedures such as in vitro fertilization can help. But even if you have no diagnosis yet, don't skip this section. There is information here that you can use.

In this section you can read about the most common methods used to treat infertility. You can learn what to expect from certain medications, what questions to ask if you are going to need surgery, how to evaluate an in vitro program. You can see how to plan a logical regimen of infertility treatment together with your doctor. Keep in mind that infertility treatment is elective—that is, it's up to you to give the go-ahead for whatever will be done. You will read here about how to consider the pros and cons of the most common treatment methods and how long to try them. Sometimes there is a completely different treatment that may give you the same odds of success, but your doctor hasn't yet suggested it to you. This section will help you to figure out, always along with the expertise of your doctor, what treatment is best for you.

Here too you will find a lot of information on coping with infertility in your emotional lives. Most couples undergoing infertility treatment have felt the great strain that comes with this experience, and you are probably no different. Here you can read about the sad things, the absurd things, and the hopeful things that happen in the lives of couples like you.

To finish up this section there is information and two essays about pregnancy after infertility. This long-awaited happy event is the goal you've long been striving for, yet still takes an adjustment. Here you'll find out that ambivalences are normal and that your great joy, happily enough, is normal too!

Do You Have a Diagnosis? Yes

You may not receive the news of your diagnosis in quite the way you've imagined. Some people have a surprising result from a workup test that suddenly takes their diagnosis in a completely new direction. Others, following a trail of clues, arrive at their logical diagnosis with no great shock.

No matter which way you receive your diagnosis, putting a name on your infertility problem is an event with great impact. You may feel as though you've been punched in the stomach—or the news might take days or weeks to sink in. Still, grasping the significance of your diagnosis and incorporating it into your life is a tough but important thing to do.

Your self images will probably take a temporary nosedive during this time. At this point, it's difficult not to feel very different from the rest of the world, and now that difference has a name—endometriosis, azoospermia, hyperprolactinemia. The names of these conditions alone can overwhelm. If you're feeling sad, strange, or depressed after hearing your diagnosis, don't be overly hard on yourself to "buck up" and be brave right away. Even if prospects for successful treatment are excellent, you need time to get used to all of this. You need a chance to adjust to the loss of normalcy that you're feeling before you resolve to fight on. And you will be very surprised at how ready you'll be to get going with your treatment.

Remember, a diagnosis isn't a death sentence. There are many, many treatable conditions under the broad umbrella of infertility, and "knowing your enemy" can fill you with the energy to conquer your problem. If you are working closely with your infertility specialist, you will be going over treatment possiblities and deciding what you can do. Just discussing treatments is a very positive, hopeful action. Allow yourself to feel sad. This feeling is natural and not uncommon. Going forward to meet your challenge can then give your life renewed purpose, a purpose that may not have been clear before you knew your diagnosis.

As you switch gears and prepare for treatments or surgery, you still may experience a variety of emotions. Some of them may be familiar to you, but at other times you will feel differently than you ever have before. Barbara Eck Menning, the founder of the organization RESOLVE and an infertility counselor for many years, has written that these feelings can be similar to the range of emotions associated with grief. The stages of emotions, originally articulated by Elisabeth Kubler-Ross, are well known to most of us but are experienced anew when dealing with infertility.

You may hear your diagnosis in disbelief—it can't be true. This feeling could be denial at work. Once the news sinks in for a while, you'll feel the unfairness of the world on your shoulders and perhaps feel great anger. You could feel resentful of the pregnant multitudes parading around in the street. Don't feel guilty about this anger, because it is very, very human and normal. Thankfully, it is temporary, too. Try not to turn this anger inward and blame yourself or each other for your infertility. Keep talking frankly and openly to one another and try to troubleshoot any anger before it becomes too serious. If you feel a rift of anger beginning to trouble your relationship, you may consider seeing a counselor for a few sessions, to get things back on a more even keel. Recognizing your anger and directing it properly is crucial, and a professional can help you do this.

Now that you have a diagnosis, you may start thinking back into your past, wondering what you did to deserve being infertile. You may come to regard infertility as a punishment. It's common to search for a cause-and-effect relationship as explanation for infertility problems. The randomness of the universe is so large and imposing that most of us have trouble accepting it. It's easier to grasp the accident of infertility as an event caused by something terrible that we ourselves have done. While this mentality can help you accept the fact of your infertility diagnosis, the acceptance is purchased at a high price. You may begin to think of yourself as a guilty person who is being punished with infertility. You may even accept infertility as something you deserve, because your "sins" have made you unworthy of fertility. This is not the case, no matter what your diagnosis says.

Working through these sad feelings is difficult, but you will eventually realize that no, you did not deserve this, and yes, you are a worthy person despite your infertility. You'll stop associating your worthiness with your infertility, and you will become itchy to begin treatment and look ahead.

But what if you have a diagnosis—and it is that your infertility is untreatable? What if you've been reading the preceding paragraphs, thinking that none of that "look-ahead-to-treatment" baloney applies to you?

You have more than just the shock of a major setback to cope with. You may feel that the door leading to the rest of your life has been slammed shut. This news is so final, so terrible, that dealing with it seems impossible right now.

If you've been told that you will not be able to conceive, carry, or give birth to your child, it will feel to you like the death of a loved one who was very close to you. In fact, it is the death of many things. It is the death of the natural, biological child you both dreamed of having. It is the death of your long-standing plans for the future. It is the end of a complete genetic attachment to your children, which right now may feel like the end of your family lineage. It's certainly the end of a level of security you once felt about living in this world. Right now it can feel like the death of hope.

For women, there may be the loss of a major part of female identity, because you will not experience childbearing. For men, an essential step toward defining manhood will not be taken. As a result, you both may feel that you are unformed, incomplete, immature, and that you will never have the opportunity to fulfill yourselves. You might start to question life's purpose; you may wonder about God's plan for you. Thinking about mortality is scarier now that you feel you've lost your link to the future.

Our culture has devised many rituals of comfort and coping for the bereaved. There are wakes, funerals, prayers, memorials, graves. Friends and family urge the grief-stricken to fully feel their grief, work it through, and begin to recover. But what happens when you lose your child who never was?

It is important for you to tell yourselves that you are entitled to grieve this loss, and to grieve fully. This was NOT a child who never was. It was a real child whom you knew well in your dreams. Accepting your diagnosis is so difficult because it means accepting the death of this child.

Grieving this death means acknowledging the child fully, then letting it go when you are able to. At this time, although comfort and support are essential, you may find little. Leaning only on each other for solace can be difficult. Learning to help each other cope with your loss is sometimes overwelming, but it is necessary if your bereavement is unknown or misunderstood by others around you.

Are there close friends or family members to whom you can turn for comfort? If you tell her you need her understanding and help, a trusted confidante can make a world of difference in your grieving process. If you can find no one, an understanding counselor or a RESOLVE contact person may be able to speak with you and let you know that you're not alone. Reaching out for this help is self-affirming and positive, even if it seems excruciatingly hard to do.

If you feel as though your grief is out of control, if you are very depressed, or if you are unable to acknowledge your loss for some reason, you may need to talk to a counselor. Counseling can also help if your loss has brought out anger in your relationship. A few sessions with a qualified professional who knows the problems of infertility can be invaluable. Remember, going to see a counselor doesn't mean you're crazy. Talking out your feelings in a controlled atmosphere away from the highly charged home front will give you a new perspective.

Most of all, you need to give yourself enough time. This news takes getting used to. Everyone needs a different amount of time, and you should not rush to pull yourself together. If you are able to fully feel your grief, it will run its course and eventually begin to lessen. This may seem impossible to believe now, but someday it will happen. The pain will never disappear, as if it never was, but do you want to completely forget this important part of your life? You will become better and better able to cope with the pain, until it is a twinge that occasionally reminds you of the love you had for your natural baby. You will be able to move beyond it, but you won't forget it.

As you begin to leave intense grief behind, you may want to start looking at the lifestyle alternatives that are available to you, and you'll wonder about the possibilities they may hold for you. You will gradually want to get on with your life, and mulling over these alternatives will help you picture what could lie ahead. Looking into different ways of building a family may be difficult at first, but it is a transition you will naturally make in your thoughts and feelings. Don't rush into any answer, but use this time as you recover from your loss as a chance to live a contemplative life, thinking new thoughts, and slowly but surely, dreaming new dreams.

Do You Have a Diagnosis? No

What if you both have been thoroughly checked, poked, prodded, and tested, but you still have no diagnosis for your infertility? In about 10 percent of cases, no concrete answer is found, and a couple is said to have unexplained infertility. Some doctors still use the bizarre term "normal infertility," which means you've tested normal, but you remain infertile. It's not fun to be told you're normal when something clearly is wrong, and "unexplained infertility" is a far more humane term for what's going on.

Terminology aside, unexplained infertility can be harder to cope with than specific bad news. Uncertainty about what's wrong can leave you puzzled and frustrated. Plus, the blank diagnosis might invite you to blame yourselves for doing something—anything—wrong, something that may have affected your fertility.

Unexplained infertility isn't mysteriously self-induced. Medical science hasn't found all the causes for this problem yet, and that may be why your answer hasn't been found. Knowing you've searched as best as you could and that you've been evaluated by knowledgeable and qualified doctors should reassure you that your problem would have been found if it could be.

Do you have an uneasy feeling that something was missed? Don't be bashful about speaking up. The logic of your workups and the results should already have been explained to you, but it could never hurt to go through it again. Ask your doctor to go over your case with you and ask any question that you might have. It's much better to blurt out a "stupid" question in the office than to lie awake at night wondering months later.

Are you wondering that you might need a second opinion? This is always a delicate subject, because you don't want to offend your doctor. Try to remember that a good doctor isn't going to be offended by your desire for another medical opinion, especially if your infertility is unexplained. The doctor is curious, too. If you have any names remaining from your original search for an infertility specialist, you can call for a second opinion. Or, you can contact your local RESOLVE and obtain a referral.

If you wish to go ahead with another medical opinion, don't do it behind your doctor's back. Be up-front. "We'd just feel better if your finding is confirmed by another specialist," is one way you can explain your reasons. Have your doctor send over a complete set of your workup records. You may want to volunteer to hand-carry them. Without even examining you, a second specialist may be able to assess your tests and corroborate your doctor's findings. Perhaps the differing point of view will cause a previously missed clue to gain importance. You won't know unless you ask.

If your current specialist is reluctant to support your desire for another opinion, this could be a warning sign. A dedicated physician interested in your welfare should not object to an evaluation made by a colleague. If your doctor strongly discourages you, be sure to find out why if you can. You may have to read between the lines. If your physician intimates that it's just your neurosis that's urging you to go elsewhere for another opinion, this is a clear signal that your emotional needs as infertility patients are being ignored. You may want to change doctors altogether if you receive too much of that kind of talk.

Only you can decide if and when a second opinion feels right. If you've had a good, open relationship with your specialist, you won't spoil it. You are the patients, the medical consumers, and this is your case. It is ultimately up to you to see that you get the medical attention that satisfies you.

Once the shock of "no diagnosis" has worn off somewhat, living month to month with unexplained infertility becomes your main challenge. The stress of this condition can alternately fill you with despair or raise your expectations high. One day you'll feel everything is hopeless, while the next you'll be sure that pregnancy is just around the corner. It's guaranteed that you'll feel both extremes, and that you'll experience these mood swings often. You aren't crazy—this is normal.

Barbara Eck Menning has compared unexplained infertility to the plight of families with soldiers who are missing in action. Menning has found through her years of counseling that couples experience an uncertainty that forces them to be simultaneously open to joyous news and prepared for terrible news. This going back and forth can be agonizing.

One solution that can help keep your life on a more even keel is to try and hold the middle ground. In her article "Infertility as a Chronic Illness," clinical psychologist Dr. Jeanne Fleming has written of one method of doing this—think of your infertility not as one sustained blow, but as a continuing condition. Compare unexplained infertility to, say, a case of arthritis or hay fever, and you'll begin to see that coping becomes a continuous activity as you wait for a more permanent solution. If you can live with infertility as an open-ended situation for the time being, you can develop methods to help you feel less panic-stricken. You can cope emotionally as well as with your medical care and with your future plans. Each is a little different, but each will greatly contribute to a more settled life right now.

For example, you probably find that family gatherings or parties that feature babies and toddlers can be particularly stressful. If you had hay fever, would you have a picnic in a ragweed field? Of course not. For the time being, you should feel no guilt about avoiding such events as a way to promote your well-being, just as you'd avoid that picnic until after hay fever season.

You may choose to keep trying to become pregnant for an indefinite period of time, or you may feel more comfortable if you begin planning to look into alternative ways of building your family. When you are feeling hopeful and optimistic, you'll be confident, but you'll also feel supported by future possibilities on the days when you're feeling disappointed. You may decide to read up about sophisticated forms of medical intervention, adoption, or even childfree living. Thinking of these alternatives as a future course of action will make your present course easier to follow, because you'll know that you have something else you can do. Talking about these alternatives now doesn't mean it's time to give up. It doesn't mean you're jinxing your chances of conception. It just means that you know you're not beaten yet.

In cases of unexplained infertility, don't drift away from your medical care. You should have a powwow with your specialist from time to time, to check in on new ideas, new tests, how you're feeling. At the very least, new semen analyses should be done every six months or so. The future of your medical treatment should be roughly planned and contingencies mapped out for you. Your doctor can steer you toward alternatives that suit you best.

Keep your plans flexible. Nobody is going to tell you to quit trying or that it's hopeless. Nobody is going to tell you that you must continue to try indefinitely. You'll probably recognize when it's time to adjust your plans. Only you can know how much uncertainty you can really cope with, and when it's time to do something else. You may find you can withstand a long period of trying because your hopes and convictions are strong. But if you find that you start to "run out of gas," you can fall back on the alternatives that you've been considering. You'll know that you did your best and that it's time for something new. With that, your hopes will renew themselves once again.

Your Infertility Treatment Is Planned

To get the clearest picture of what's happening with your case, distinguish in your minds the difference between testing and treatment for infertility. Your workups uncovered the problem. Now you must decide with your specialist what to do about it.

You've probably been tested for most of the known conditions that contribute to infertility. When you are diagnosed, the doctor will begin to recommend a course of action, such as a program of drug therapy, corrective surgery, perhaps a change in your lovemaking practices, or any combination of these. Be sure you understand your diagnosis. Be sure you are thoroughly briefed on how and why a certain treatment is right for you. Only then can you make intelligent decisions and participate fully with your doctor.

The timetable of tests followed by treatments is not the same for any two patients. Treatment for minor ovulation problems, for example, could commence before all your workup tests are complete. This is the smart way to save time. Just be sure one minor problem doesn't bring all investigation to a halt before the full picture for your case is apparent.

Having a plan for your infertility treatment, discussed and agreed upon between you and your doctor, is essential. A meeting of the minds about what lies ahead is a foundation for understanding and promotes good morale for you as patients. This plan will give you a feeling of control you may have missed up to now. It will keep up your confidence in your physician and maintain open communication all around. You won't feel like you're walking ahead into unknown territory. Your plan will help you know what to expect, and it will give you an approximate time frame. It provides alternatives to treatments, too. If one treatment doesn't seem to work, you know you can try something else.

The plan you make together doesn't have to be absolute. It is a guideline. It isn't an achievement test for either you or your doctor. It is a set of realistic expectations worked out according to your individual case. There will always be room for extra tries, new treatment breakthroughs, even miracles. The plan helps direct you step-by-step, that's all.

You and your doctor should have an in-office consultation, which, if preferred, could be separate from a medical visit. Be sure to come together for this meeting, no matter who is being treated. If you have a lot of questions, this is the time to ask them. Be sure you will have enough time to talk, so let the receptionist and the doctor know that you need time for a thorough discussion of your case.

As treatments are explained to you, the doctor will naturally explain them in terms of a successful outcome. Great . But it may be up to you to ask, "What do we do if this doesn't work?" As you hear your doctor's answer, you'll hear your treatment plan begin to emerge.

You must plan together. Tell your doctor your special needs, consider your ages, talk about how much time you'll need. What is your goal? Does this treatment move you toward this goal? Are the risks and inconveniences worth the odds of success that you gain?

Be realistic if you can. Successful treatment of a problem may not insure pregnancy, but only enhanced chances for a pregnancy. Be sure both you and your doctor are speaking the same language.

Here are questions you may want to ask about your proposed treatment:

Questions to Ask About a Proposed Treatment

- What treatment do you propose? Why does that suit our case?
- Does this involve medication, surgery, or something else?
- What will this do to correct the problem?
- What are the chances that this will work?
- If it works, what are our odds of pregnancy?
- How long should we give this treatment?
- When will we know if it is working? How will we know?
- How much will it cost?

- Is it painful?
- Are there any risks?
- Are there side effects?
- Does this treatment interfere with any other medication?
- Will this interfere with moods, make me nervous, affect sexual drive, vision, reflexes, etc.?
- Is there any other way to treat this problem?
- Can we use the second method if the first method doesn't work?
- What are the particulars of the alternative treatment?
- Will treatment interfere with daily life?
- Are you experienced in administering this treatment?
- How is treatment monitored?
- Will we be referred to receive this treatment? To whom?
- If we are referred will you follow up closely?
- Is this treatment considered experimental by doctors?
- Do you know if this treatment is considered experimental by insurers?
- Is this treatment usually covered by insurers?
- Are there any hidden expenses to this treatment?
- What do we do if this doesn't work?

Many common fertility problems have well agreed-upon treatments that your doctor will fine-tune to suit your case. But this doesn't mean you are obligated to accept your treatment blindly. Read about it, ask about it, call RESOLVE about it, and be sure you have all the facts, and that you and your doctor are both up to date.

Some treatments involve corrective surgery. If surgery is suggested for you, here are some questions you may want to ask:

Questions to Ask If you Need Surgery
- Have we done everything possible to avoid surgery?
- Can we avoid general anesthesia and still have comfortable, effective surgery?
- Who will be my surgeon? Can I speak to the surgeon in advance?

- I'd like time to obtain a second opinion. Is there any problem with that?

Here are some questions for the surgeon:

- What is your surgical training?
- What is the extent of your experience?
- What is your success rate in surgeries of this type?
- What scar will I be left with?
- What surgical techniques do you plan to use?
- Do you practice microsurgical techniques whenever possible?
- Are you trained in laser surgery?
- Can I talk to a past patient of yours with my problem?
- Do I need to be admitted to the hospital? How long will I be in?
- What anesthetic will be used?
- What effects can I expect from it?
- What are the risks associated with this surgery?
- What are the costs? Your fee? Anesthesiologist's fee? OR (operating room) fees?
- What pre-op tests do I need?
- Is this surgery considered experimental by doctors or insurers?
- Is this surgery covered by insurance?
- What are the side effects of this surgery?
- Pain?
- How long will I need to recover?
- When can I resume normal activities?
- Do I need to take time off from work?
- When will we know if surgery was a success? How will we know?
- Do you personally follow up?
- Will I need any medication following surgery?
- Will I feel differently afterwards?
- Can I put this off and try something else first?

- Is the benefit worth any possible risk?
- What is the pregnancy rate for others with this problem who have had surgery?
- What if this doesn't work? What can we do?
- Can I bank my own blood in advance?
- Will there be a videotaped record of this surgery?
- Do you communicate directly with my doctor to give results?

If surgery has been recommended, it is common practice for the patient to obtain a second opinion. This second opinion will not offend or threaten your doctor, so don't feel bashful if you'd like one. Especially in cases of infertility, there are advances being made all the time that might help you to avoid major surgery, and you need to find out all the facts available to you. Getting a second opinion will help you be sure you know everything.

When you have a clear picture of what your treatment involves, you can decide if it's what you want and need right now. Don't forget, most infertility treatment is elective—this means that there's no illness or medical emergency involved. You must decide positively that this is for you. Knowing as much as you can gives you the freedom to make the best decisions possible. Your plan for treatment will have no surprises, and you will feel secure and confident that you're on the right track.

Reassessing Your Treatment

In a perfect world you'd have the perfect specialist who treats you as an intelligent couple, who has plenty of time, infinite wisdom, low fees, no other patients, is totally honest yet compassionate, has a convenient location, and completely understands your emotional as well as physical difficulties.

During your months of treatment for infertility, it's easy to focus on your doctor as a powerful person who is able to cure you. Shifting all this power and responsibility to the doctor can relieve you of your burden of worries, but doing so may catch up with you later. Stay involved yourself, even if you are sick of this subject. Realize that your doctor is human, and that infertility is a continually evolving specialty. More remains to be learned by both you and your doctor. If you have a treatment plan in mind, you can remind yourselves periodically of your timetable, and ready yourselves to switch treatments if necessary. Work with your doctor in monitoring your progress and keep a handle on how you're doing.

Impatience and frustration, teamed up with poor doctor-patient communication, causes patients to leave their infertility specialists every day. If you are tracking your case in tandem with your doctor, you can go far in avoiding this problem. Following your case will keep you thinking realistically, it will stop you from panicking, and it will keep your doctor from looming before you as an all-powerful, distant figure. It will prevent you from leaving competent medical care for the wrong reasons.

But there are instances when leaving for a new specialist is a good idea. You are looking for two things from your doctor: compassionate service and results. If you are dissatisfied with one or the other, and you feel you have legitimate, logical reasons, you should consider changing physicians and not feel guilty.

Ask yourself some of these questions:

- Is our treatment going along pretty closely to the plans?
- Are we being carefully monitored?
- Do we still feel we are moving positively towards our goal? Or is this starting to feel like it's taking too long?
- Does our doctor handle our questions and problems promptly, seriously, frankly, humanely?
- Do we feel secure with our doctor's skills?
- Does our doctor give us reassurances based on facts?
- Are we given the pertinent information that we need?
- Are our emotional needs acknowledged?
- Do lab results come back promptly? Do we receive them quickly, and are they explained thoroughly?
- Are we seeing the doctor's assistant or an associate too often?
- Do we wait too long in the reception area?
- Are the prices just too high?
- Is the support staff treating us well?
- Does our doctor seem "stuck" on one treatment idea?
- Does the doctor order excessive and expensive tests?
- Does the doctor know our case without prompting from us?

- Can we trust our doctor to know when it's time to try something else?
- Do we look forward to or dread our appointments?

If you are considering leaving your current doctor, you may feel tempted to avoid a confrontation and simply disappear. At the very least you will need your records forwarded, so this is a bad idea. Plus, you should want your doctor to know why you are leaving so that the service given to future patients will improve. If you feel strongly that you have been ill-served, you must be heard, in case there is a serious misunderstanding interfering with your medical care.

You can speak to the doctor over the phone, if possible, or you can put your thoughts in writing. Be clear about your reasons, and be as logical as you can be. If in the end you simply have a problem with your doctor's manner that you can no longer live with, you can merely state that you have decided to seek alternate care. You can indicate that your emotional needs were not well served, but that you do feel you received skillful medical attention. You don't have to elaborate unless you want to.

When you begin seeing a new specialist, you can't relax just yet. You need to hear a new opinion of your case and find out if your treatment is going to change. Your plans may have to be redrawn drastically. You should explain why you left your last doctor, and what you feel you need now. A compassionate, professional physician will appreciate your frankness.

Infertility in Everyday Living

If Only One of You Is Being Treated

Infertility is a medical problem that involves two people. It takes two to make a baby. Even if only one person needs medical treatment, you both remain directly involved.

Still, if you are the person with the problem, you may feel guilt, sadness, and even fear of rejection. You need time to regain your equilibrium and feel secure in your relationship. You also need to come to grips with your partner's feelings. Orchestrating your emotional needs as individuals, then working on your commitment together takes time and lots of talking. It can be done, though, and you can do it.

Attending important medical appointments together helps give support and is worth the time and effort it takes. It can be lonely and frightening to face a string of appointments alone, and this could contribute to feelings of resentment.

Even if time off from the job is necessary, try to present a united front at the doctor's.

If you are being treated and feel overstressed at being the only one who is poked and prodded, you're bound to express it sooner or later. When you need to blow off some of these feelings, avoid blaming your partner. Rage at fate instead. Chances are your spouse would give anything to turn the tables and take this burden from you.

If you are the partner who is not being treated, you may feel strange about getting off "free." Don't feel guilty about this, and don't feel guilty if your partner's infertility is upsetting you. It is terrible. You are entitled to be upset. But feeling upset and giving needless blame are two different things. It's a delicate balance, but you must try to support your spouse and acknowledge your own feelings, too.

You won't be able to help each other with just a snap of your fingers, but together you can create an emotional refuge that can be a source of comfort. Listen to each other, talk to each other. Ask one another, "How are you feeling today?" Be honest. Give the other the right to feel differently than you do. If you are going to disagree and you're going to fight about it, try to keep your heads and fight fairly. No recriminations allowed.

If you are having a lot of trouble getting along, don't panic. Infertility has a way of drawing out a couple's differences and emphasizing them. You will find out things about each other that you never knew before, both good and bad. This can only help you forge a better, stronger relationship, but it is pretty difficult to live through day by day. If you think you need help sorting things out, you can take a break from treatment, or you can consider going to counseling. All you may need are instructions on how to have a productive fight. Or you may find that counseling can open up new ways of communication in all areas of your relationship. If you have not hesitated to obtain medical help, don't balk if you suspect you also need a little help with the emotional burden you're carrying.

Life on "Hold"

Have you ever made an important phone call and been put on hold? The maddening frustration of infertility can feel like you've been put on hold in all parts of your life. You may feel you cannot make any concrete plans for your future, because you don't know what lies ahead. Should you take that promotion at the office? Should you buy that house you planned for? Sometimes a woman can't even buy clothes without wondering what shape she'll be in later.

Being in limbo due to infertility can often affect how we judge ourselves in our other life achievements. Are we growing and changing, building our lives, reaching maturity? We often use childbearing as a yardstick of adulthood, and infertility can make us feel we've fallen short of the mark.

In your minds, try to separate infertility from other important aspects of your life. You may have to sternly talk some sense into yourselves. Recognize societal standards and pressures as artificial constructs, and remember that you are a worthy person regardless of the way you meet these standards. The fact that you are having trouble getting pregnant isn't a brand that stamps you as incompetent. It is a medical problem that you are taking care of.

Avoid thinking that actions in other parts of your life will or won't affect your prospects of pregnancy. If you are considering taking on more responsibility at work, you may fear that a surprise pregnancy would prevent you from doing a good job. Is that really your fear? Or do you fear the extra work will somehow prevent pregnancy? Try to be clear on your motives. Consider a career move on its own merits, not in light of your reproductive plans. Do you need the money? Do you want the job? Is it a move up? Will the stress in your life increase? Will this job bolster your self-esteem at a time when you need it? Will it be an important distraction from your problems? Let these practical considerations lead your thinking. Becoming pregnant after a promotion will be a happy complication in your life, and solving that problem will be easier than solving infertility.

Some people put off moving to a new home because they feel that a delayed pregnancy means they don't need it. Or is it because they now feel that they don't deserve it? Putting off nest-building in this way could make you feel even more deprived than you're feeling now. Or you might feel that having those extra unoccupied rooms will emphasize your misery.

Try not to dwell on the extra bedrooms as symbols of infertility and think about why other people move into roomier living quarters. Don't you also want a better kitchen? More storage space? To live in a better neighborhood? The happy challenge of fixing up a house? These are also wonderful and worthy reasons to move. Balance out your feelings and talk it over. Think of your future home not as a reward for fertility but as something you do to improve your life.

You can apply this type of thinking to other major decisions you may face while you're waiting to conceive. You don't have to put your entire life on hold. You can make rational decisions about going back to school, joining a professional organization, taking on volunteer duties in your community, bringing home a pet.

Don't make pregnancy the only green light in your life. You have the power to succeed at many other tasks of living, and you should not neglect them now

Surely THIS Will Be the Month

KATIE GEORGE

i have a "normal" routine I go through every month while my husband and I are trying to conceive a baby. Some people refer to the monthly cycle as the emotional roller coaster, but I'd call my routine a depression-go-round.

The first day of the cycle is, of course, the first day of my period. Sometimes I am expecting it, having felt bleak and pessimistic after reading my body signs correctly: swelled breasts, a low ache in the abdomen, a quick temper. When the blood finally appears, it's just the last nail in the coffin. These are the months when I just become numb during the first day of my period—no hysterics, just grim acceptance of fate. It was not to be.

These are the times when I punish myself for daring to hope. You thought you might like a baby? What gave you such a notion? I actually delay taking my Motrin tablet and let my menstrual cramps grip me. After all, I deserve to feel physical as well as emotional pain, right?

A few hours later, of course, I run to the medicine cabinet and gulp down the Motrin—the pain is beginning to bring me to my senses. For the zillionth time I wonder if these bad cramps could mean endometriosis. Can I trust my doctor's assessment of my laparoscopy?

As my period nears its end, I take up the temperature regimen with fresh zeal. This will be the month. No more of this nonsense. We'll take the readings correctly, I'll watch my cervical mucus, we'll hit the right day, and all will be well at last.

Around Day 7 or 8 my husband and I discuss when we should get on the schedule, that is, when do we start our every-forty-eight-hours rendezvous routine? We decide that this month we'll go with Days 9, 11, 13, 15, and surely that will do it. Since I can't stand those urine tests every month, this is our way to be sure.

So we make love and tick off the days. The thermometer becomes a powerful master in the middle of the month. Will we get in just one more "session" before the reading jumps, indicating ovulation has ocurred? Sometimes the timing is way off or we miss a chance, and the damned thing goes up before we're ready for it to. Ka-phlooey. But this month we've pulled it off beautifully. There goes the mercury, right on schedule. We did it.

When we feel that we've done everything as right as we can, we dare to allow ourselves to be filled with hope. This could be it. This is the enjoyable part of the month. For one thing, if we're sick of sex, we take a break. But mostly, we feel a new sense of purpose—we might be expecting a baby. For these last two weeks I usually switch from aspirin to Tylenol, go with decaf coffee, skip the wine. Doesn't it sound nutty? I guess I'm just making sacrifices, however small and symbolic, for this hoped-for pregnancy. If this is it, I'll never ingest the wrong foods again, I promise.

I start listening to my body with great concentration. What was that twinge? Mittelschmerz is unknown to me, but I will not let any other sign go by unnoticed. Why am I tired today? Is this really a stomach ache? I argue against my common sense. Gee, my breasts are sore—wait, they're always a little sore at about this time. But this month, they're much more sensitive—or are they?

A few days before my cycle is due to wind up, my optimism is tempered with fear. What if I did conceive, but it didn't implant? Should I really be roughhousing like this? I know it's all silly, but what if just one tiny thing goes wrong that I could have controlled?

Then I start feeling those funny flowing sensations. Oh no—is this it? I keep running to the bathroom to check. I even do the Q-tip test. Insert a Q-tip halfway into the vagina to see if any blood is traveling down. So far I pass, so far I pass.

I wake up the next day and slide the thermometer into my mouth. Five minutes tick by, but, wait, it's not finished yet. Back into the mouth. A little rub of the tongue—that's cheating, I know. My hormones don't know what my tongue is doing, and they have their own agenda. Seven minutes. The temp is still down.

It has dropped. That's it. I can't quite believe it's happened again. Not this time. We did everything right. But my temperature indeed has fallen and my period will come today.

These are the months that I get very upset. This is NOT fair. What do we have to do, God? These are the months I cry.

Then, I dry my tears and start again. I number my next temperature chart, and put it by the bed. Surely, THIS will be the month....

Everybody's Pregnant but Us!

Everyday living with infertility tests and treatments is stressful enough. But take a walk down any residential street or go to any shopping mall and what do you see? Families, families, families. Pregnant bellies out to here. Infants in strollers. Proud papas and beaming mamas. Everybody else in the world is flaunting their happiness in your face.

Often it's easy to assume you're the only two miserable people in the world. It seems everybody can get pregnant but you. Going out just to run an errand becomes a reminder of your condition. You might even consider staying home just to avoid the passing parade of fertility going by.

Your sensitivity to this subject could be distorting your perspective. It might be painful, but do go out and try to be observant. Not everybody is pregnant; it's just that you're tuned in to seeing pregnancy now. And is it really true that all those mommies and daddies are beaming with absolute happiness, or is that your envy talking? If you look carefully you'll see tired parents, yowling children, broken toys, tear-stained cheeks as well as the blissfully happy.

Remind yourselves of the statistics. Many couples have infertility problems. You are not a strange minority with a bizarre, exotic problem, even though there are days when that's how you feel. Fifteen to 20 percent of all couples have trouble getting pregnant. You aren't the only ones, even in a family-oriented shopping mall.

If you stay home, the spectacle of the ideal, happy family is beamed at you via television, on radio, in magazines. Advertising is the worst offender. Ads for Pampers seem designed to make infertiles lose it. But even commercials for products completely unrelated to babies use them to make a sale. Whether it's tires, cameras, dog food, or soft drinks, you see commercials all day long that remind you that you don't have your baby yet.

Don't let them get to you. Don't fall apart—get cynical instead. Advertisers and television writers resort to emotional appeals when they're out of ideas. They exploit chubby babies just to get our attention, and it usually works. When there's nothing good to say about the product, they trot out the infants. It's uncreative. Don't buy into it.

The fuss in the press when a public figure gives birth can rankle, too. Just going through the supermarket line is impossible without seeing magazines and newspapers featuring the latest celebrity mom. But, just like those advertisements, these magazines are trying to make a sale. Everybody responds, even a little, to these emotional appeals, and in that second, the publisher hopes the

YOUR INFERTILITY TREATMENT 135

consumer will grab the magazine and buy it. Recognize these stress-inducing manipulations for what they are, and direct your attention to the candy display or study your shopping list. It takes practice to stop feeling victimized, but you can do it.

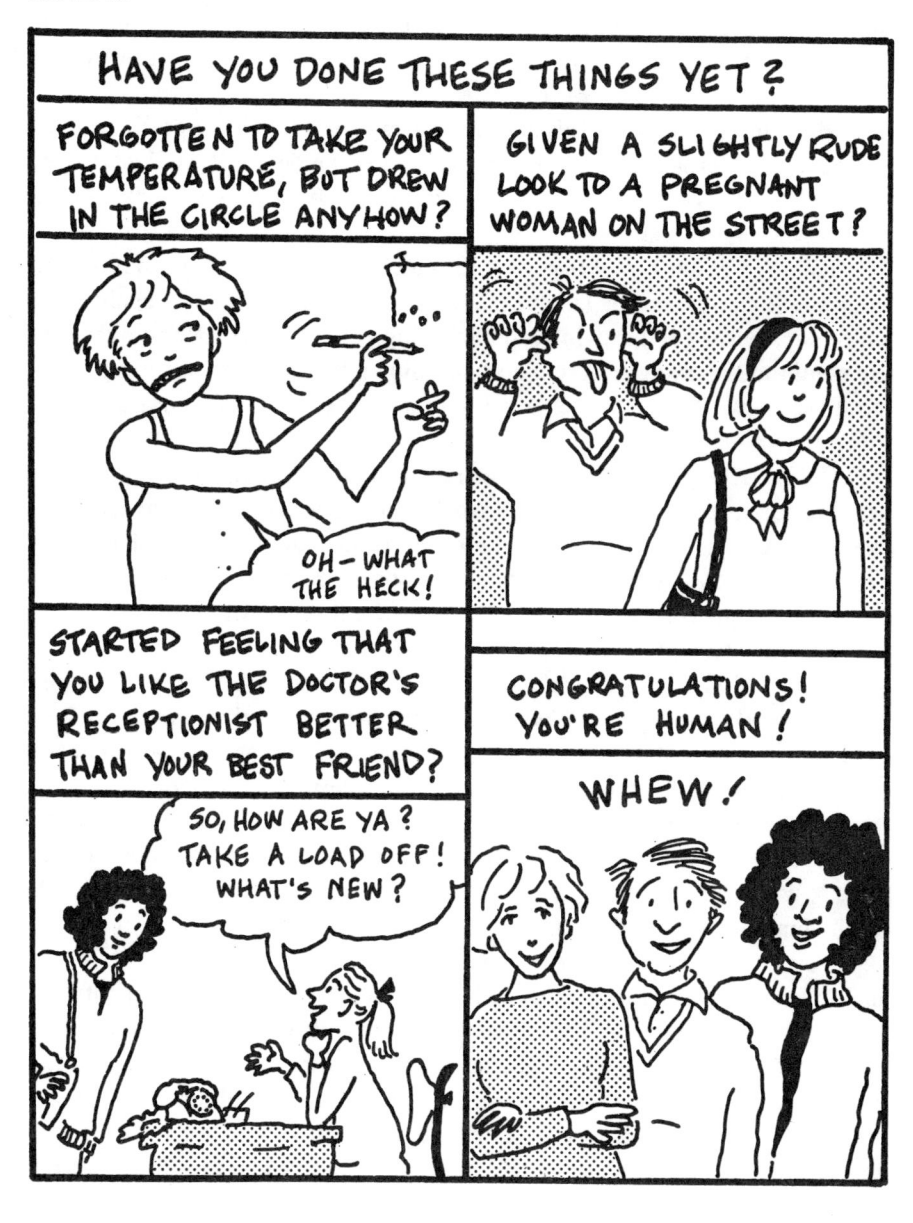

At Home: Talking and Not Talking

Every day you are reminded of infertility because you must take your temperature, you have a pill to swallow, you have a shot to take. Or, you're invited to a baby shower, your cousin with the twin toddlers is having a barbecue, or the queen of England has a new grandchild. There's just no getting away from it.

Many of us respond to this constant barrage of reminders by talking about it. Some of us verbalize our annoyances, worries, anxieties. We talk about our fears before they can come true. Talking about our frustrations seems to be the only way to let off steam.

Talking's good, right? If you're not much of a talker, you probably don't think so. Sometimes talking about the same problem over and over again, every single day, drives you batty instead of making you feel better. Non-talkers find the continuous assault of verbalizing not only irritating, but it causes them to close themselves off in defense. Other non-talkers seem to think not mentioning this problem may help it go away.

Unfortunately, lots of couples facing infertility are comprised of one talker and one non-talker. While one person feels a strong need to discuss, analyze, and speculate aloud, the other person may be turned off by this activity. This opposition of coping skills can escalate into a breakdown of much-needed communication. One partner feels the loss of a listener, while the other feels beseiged. What to do?

Family counselors and professionals experienced in helping infertile couples are familiar with this pattern. Regulating the communication habits you have fallen into can be a challenge, but if both partners are willing, you can take some important steps to change how you talk about infertility together.

Merle Bombardieri, a social worker who has counseled and written extensively on infertility, has suggested a method called the "The Twenty-Minute Rule." With this technique, couples can equalize their contributions to the discussion of infertility, and confine this discussion to a special part of the day.

You must agree together to work on this. Both of you will gain, so that should be an incentive if one of you is reluctant. In order to get infertility into better perspective in your life, agree to talk about it for only a short period of time, once a day. Each person will have the same amount of time (say, twenty minutes each) to speak up, complain, fret, speculate, cry, solve a problem. The person who usually talks too much will be forced to articulate more efficiently and talk less. The person who clams up will be forced to talk more, getting feelings out into the open. Each partner must listen carefully to the other.

Confining infertility conversation to a specific time can help you cease dwelling on it all day. You can tell yourself, "I'll talk about it later," much as Scarlett O'Hara decided she'd "think about it tomorrow." Knowing you will finally have the full attention of your partner may be all the support you need. You'll now have time to actually talk about other things—how the baseball team did, that awful new popular song, your crazy neighbor. Small talk can be such a relief sometimes, and now you can be free to indulge in some.

If you have had a particularly bad day, if you've just gotten some bad news, or if you are distressed more than normal, the rigidity of the rule can certainly be relaxed. The pressure of talking only twenty minutes after hearing you need more surgery is certainly going to overwhelm you, so don't be slavish about adhering to your guidelines. The Twenty-Minute Rule is to help you on the ordinary, run-of-the-mill days of infertility that we all have, not for periods of crisis.

What if you feel overflowing with emotion every day, and need far more than twenty or thirty minutes to express your feelings? One wonderful solution to this is to write them down. Write letters to yourself or keep a diary.

You could find that a journal is a friend with an unending capacity to listen. A journal will never tell your secrets, chide you for being silly, or judge you. You can freely express anger, jealousy, depression, even those flashes of hatred we can be so ashamed of feeling. By writing out your experiences and feelings, you'll learn new things about yourself and gain perspective. Someday, when all this is over, you can either cherish your journal as a poignant document of your struggle, or you can throw it into the fireplace.

You don't have to be a best-selling author or the perfect speller to try this. Just set down what you're feeling. Don't be afraid to express yourself; really stretch. You don't have to write into your journal regularly if you don't feel like it, but it will be there when you need to blow off steam. Even in the middle of the night, you'll have a way to channel your nervous energy and vent your feelings. Consider trying it—you might get hooked.

Talking About Infertility with Others

Incorporating infertility into daily life, however temporarily, includes deciding which people should know what's happening to you. When you're going through workups and being treated for a problem, your daily schedule, your social life, your moods can all change. The expenses of infertility can cause you to change your spending habits. You two may have started keeping more to yourselves than you used to do. People close to you have probably noticed that things with you are somehow different.

It's natural to want to tell people what's going on, but to also be afraid of telling. It helps to think in advance about whom you'd like to tell and how much you want them to know. You have the right to say however much or little you feel is necessary. If a nosy relative is likely to blab your personal problems all over the neighborhood, don't feel bad about keeping details to yourself. If a friend has shown understanding toward you in the past, you may want to spend some time talking about your infertility more extensively.

What do you need in return? The prospect of telling something so personal can scare some people. What will your listener say or do? You can minimize the risk of being "burned" by preparing to help your friends and relatives give you what you need. It's a fact that no one is a mind reader, and you must accept the added chore of helping others to help you. If you want to be taken seriously, indicate to your listener how important this conversation is to you, and don't have it at the bus stop. If you don't want to be prompted by questions about your progress, say thanks for the concern, but you will let them know when you have any news. Until that day, please, no more questions. If your listener becomes very involved with your situation and wants to know more, you've hit the jackpot. Help them learn, just as you've helped yourself learn. There is special literature for family members and friends of infertile people that they might find very helpful. Give them *Understanding—A Guide to Impaired Fertility for Family and Friends,* by Patricia I. Johnston (available from Perspectives Press), and let them read your medical books.

No matter how carefully you explain what's happening and what you need, some people just aren't going to catch on. The pain of infertility can seem to double when it's being discussed by an insensitive friend or relative. Everybody has "horror stories" of inapproprite or cruel remarks, awkward situations, or embarrassments. They happen in other parts of your life, and they will happen in connection with infertility, too.

You might feel deeply wounded, righteously indignant, or just plain mad when these "horrors" happen. How can people be so dumb? So mean? Why do they carry on this way?? What is wrong with them??

Do not take responsibility for the actions of these people. Ultimately, their behavior is their problem, not your problem. It's THEIR problem. Repeat it to yourself firmly and slowly. It's the truth.

The fact is, some people are clods. Even people you love. You can still love them. But separate their remarks or behavior from the rest of their personality if you possibly can. It's difficult and it takes time, but it can be done. These folks may have a short attention span for a problem that can trouble you for months or years. After a while, they just tune out—they simply can't pay attention any longer. Some people cannot empathize with a problem they don't have themselves. Infertility doesn't compute in their data banks, so they just don't know what to do or say. Some people are frightened or threatened by such a fundamental adversity, and this fear might be expressed in how you are treated. If you can, show your strength in fighting infertility, that you are not diminished by the battle.

Finally, some people just say the wrong things, even if they are given pointers and advice. Short of holding up cue cards for these folks, there's not much you can do to change them. Don't expend a lot of energy wondering why you can't get through to them. It's their problem, remember?

Want to Know a Secret?

CAROL PETERS

I don't believe there is a graceful segue into the subject of infertility. Can you bring it up between the entrée and dessert? No, too involved. How about practicing on your hairdresser? Mine is eight months pregnant. Does this seem like someone who would understand infertility? Begin at the beginning, perhaps. Tell the family? Mine, to a person, still blurts out thoughtless questions and ridiculous clichés, even though they know how desperately we are trying to conceive a child.

The only advice I can give someone experiencing infertility is don't tell anyone until you have adjusted to the problem yourself. If others wonder out loud about your plans for a family, just smile like the Cheshire cat and disappear. When you have found that you are able to deal with your problem emotionally, tell those you feel must know.

But don't feel pressured into explaining yourself or your life to anyone. As you become more open about your infertility, however, you will discover that you will occasionally stike harmonious chords with others. People you may never have suspected of being infertile will nod and say yes, we understand what you are going through. These sympathetic moments will more than compensate for any awkwardness you may experience with less sensitive people.

Everyone I have known who has experienced infertility has found it difficult to impossible to explain the situation to family or friends. My family behaves as if I'm working on a construction project. Despite all the delays, the building will be finished.

Everyone handles this situation differently. It took me over a year to become comfortable with talking about my condition and the status of my infertility. However, I don't tell my family when I begin and end a cycle of medical treatment. If I do, they call me to either express condolences or ask personal questions—additional stress when I need it least.

So, my advice is know thyself. And listen to the voice in your head that tells you, "It's time." Then do your best.

Protecting Yourself

Just as you must be realistic in your expectations of friends and relatives, be equally realistic in what you expect from yourself. Just as you accept the shortcomings of others, accept your own without self-recriminations.

One of the ways some couples with infertility problems "test" themselves is by enduring social situations that can be excruciatingly painful. Attending and smiling through baby showers is an obvious example, but family reunions, holiday parties, and neighborhood barbecues can also qualify.

It's nice to be invited. It's better to be invited than to be deliberately excluded in plans made by friends and relatives. Be sure those around you know you'd like to be remembered and how much you appreciate being asked. Tell them to keep asking. But if you particularly dread an event because you know pregnancy or children will be a central focus, you have a right to say no. What will you have proved if you're miserable before this event, during it, and for hours afterward?

Social gatherings are supposed to be fun, so unless the odds are good that you will indeed enjoy yourself, think about making alternative plans—and feel no guilt. Don't use a kiddie birthday party as a trial by fire, in hopes that surviving this agony marks you as truly deserving of pregnancy. Pregnancy doesn't work that way. Don't deliberately increase the difficulty of your situation; it's difficult enough.

You will not become a hermit if you turn down some well-chosen invitations or miss a family party. A time will come when you'll look forward to these events again, and you'll go and enjoy yourselves.

In the meantime, try to anticipate situations that you may find hard to get through, and decide if they are important enough for you to go to. If not, skip them. Especially during the winter holidays, you may face a string of gatherings that will try your emotions. Pick and choose the best ones for you to attend, and plan personal time together in substitution for the rest. It's not chicken-hearted to avoid extra pain. It's a gesture of love and nurturing just for yourselves.

If you simply can't get out of something, rehearse yourself in the privacy of your bathroom. Look into the mirror and practice comebacks to various questions and remarks you may hear. After it's over, reward yourselves with a gallon of ice cream or a nice massage. You did it!

The quality of your life right now is just as important as your future family. You do have the right to protect yourselves from unnecessary stress and pain with no apology. Be glad you are able to recognize what you need and that you are able to act accordingly. It's a great self-preservation skill.

If a Close Friend Gets Pregnant

When a close friend comes to you with exciting news of her pregnancy, it can be devastating. The strangers you see out in the street are a mere abstraction, but when a loving friend or family member gets pregnant, infertility can become even harder to bear.

In this situation, our emotions can literally go to war. Yes, of course we are happy for them, and we congratulate them heartily. Then, we feel intensely jealous. A momentary flash of hatred, impossible as it seems, may even show itself. Then of course, we feel guilty for harboring such negative feelings for someone we love so much.

All these feelings are normal and very human. Watching someone else grow more pregnant every day, and sharing in it as close friends often do, is very difficult for most of us. Forgive yourself for your shortcomings. You can only do the best you can.

Does your friend understand about your infertility? If so, she may feel a little guilty exulting in front of you. If she does not know, you must decide if telling her is something you should do. Choose a time and place when her pregnancy isn't in the conversation, and let her know your situation. An honest and heartfelt explanation now will save misunderstandings later if you cannot bring yourself to throw a shower or visit her in the hospital. Your good friend will try to understand. Trust her. Then you can relax and be genuinely happy for her.

Philosophical and Religious Consideration

Couples dealing with infertility grapple with more than doctors, tests, or hospitals. Often we have to face those larger questions about life that perhaps we hadn't thought much about in the past. Questions, doubts, and despair can sometimes threaten our outlook on life. If we have been religious in the past, we need to redefine our faith. If we don't follow an organized religion, we may develop a bond with God for the first time. At the very least, we all become philosophers.

The ability to readily become pregnant, bear children, and rear a family is so basic, so fundamental, that few of us give thought to what may go wrong with our plans. Then we discover that it's not so easy. We start to wonder what all of this could possibly mean. We start trying to answer questions that have traditionally stumped the greatest thinkers. The biggest problems of the universe suddenly seem to apply to us, and this is frightening.

Some of the questions that can keep us awake include:

- Why did this happen?
- Is this what we deserve?
- Why is it so easy for others but not us?
- What is life's purpose, if not to procreate?
- Can we be complete without children?
- What is my identity if not as a parent?
- Why do we want children anyway?
- Will this suffering make me a better person?
- Why does this hurt so much?
- Did this strike us at random?
- Can two people be a family?
- Is my commitment to my partner enough?

Experts such as psychologists, the clergy, and medical specialists have all made attempts to explain the intense feelings that can be associated with infertility. In the end, we all must work out our own version of the answers in order to live at peace with this problem.

Many feel that extra guidance is very helpful, and some seek it through religion. Others need a more secular perspective. You should not turn away from your need to question, for it too is a way to overcome infertility. Your body, your emotions, and your spirit all need attention right now.

Reading about the philosophical aspects of adversity can give you a fresh point of view. RESOLVE offers many articles that can help you work out your questions. Books abound on the subject of overcoming adversity, though few deal directly with the problem of infertility. There is a universality about the pain you are feeling, and you may be able to gain help from any number of books available that appear at first to be completely unrelated. (See the Appendix for some books to read.)

Many of us do express our deepest feelings about life through religious faith. Infertility can shake up even a devout believer, or it can draw us closer to God. As we think about what has happened in light of religion, we might ask these questions:

- Did God choose me for infertility? Why?

- Is God all-powerful? If so, why is suffering allowed to exist? If not, what is the purpose of worshiping God?
- Who is God to me now? Has my faith changed?
- What can God do to help me? What should I ask for?
- How can I know God's purpose for me?
- Am I angry at God? Do I dare express this anger?
- Am I afraid of losing faith?
- Does God love me? Do I love God?
- Do I need God the same way as before?
- How much strength does God ask of me?
- What is a miracle? Does God provide it?

It seems obvious that we can use our faith as a comfort, as an explanation of the world, as a way to pray for children. But are babies what we ought to be praying for? Rather than just asking for a child, ask in your prayers to receive strength, patience, compassion, understanding, wisdom. These are the prayers that surely will be answered.

Have you talked to your minister, priest, or rabbi? Does your pastor show insight into the particular problems of infertility? If you feel you aren't being properly heard, consider that this may be a new counseling problem for him or her. If you wish to speak openly and deeply, you may have to help out by recommending some literature or by debunking the usual myths about infertility. Just as you once had mistaken ideas about infertility, so might your pastor. If you straighten out your pastor's misconceptions, you'll be helping other couples who seek similar help in the future.

If your religion restricts how you may be treated for infertility, you may find that what your doctor prescribes is what your faith forbids. There is no easy solution for you if you feel you must choose between your religion and having a family. This crisis is a very personal one. You may be able to speak to a leader of your faith who has less restrictive views and hear how others have worked out this problem. You may choose to break from your religion. Or you may find a deeper faith in following the instructions your religion shows you.

Try to give yourselves time. If you allow yourselves the chance, quiet prayer and contemplation eventually help bring insight, strength, and the ability to recognize what you should do.

I Often Ask Myself

LISA HARRIS

i often ask myself what I'll do if I don't have children. Where will life take me if I don't stop along the way to change a diaper, tie a shoe, or go to a school play? Whom will I watch fall in love or out of love? Who will come to me and want to know about the things I did as a child? Was I ever scared? Did I ever have a failed friendship? Did the boys tease me?

There are so many things I want to tell my children. I love you. Be nice to people. Try to help those who are less fortunate. I love you. You can do anything you want with determination and grit. I'll always love you, no matter what. Let's go for a picnic, a bike ride. Let's make a surprise for Daddy.

I just hope and pray with all my heart that I will have children to say these things to.

If He'd Just Let Me Get Pregnant

MARY SHIELDS ROSS

*i*f you believe in God, there is a certain amount of bargaining involved with infertility. I have actually caught myself saying, "If He'd just let me get pregnant, I'll gladly carry through July and August. I won't complain about being hot and swollen." This may sound ridiculous coming from an intelligent, educated woman. However, infertility can rid you of the ability to rationalize on even the lowest level. It's OK to bargain with God. It doesn't seem to work, but it's still OK. Perhaps it would be better just to ask God to give me the strength to get through the whole ordeal. I really would like to make it through with my body and sanity intact.

Taking a Break

Are you becoming weary of the infertility routine? As months wear on, this happens to many couples. If you'd like to bolster your strength to keep on trying, you might consider taking a break for a cycle or two (or more) so you can catch your breath.

Sound unthinkable? If you are like most couples, the idea of missing even one month is the very opposite of what you've been trying to do. Any month might be the Fateful One. To miss several deliberately would be nuts.

But what is your true goal? Your goal is also to keep your life as comfortable as possible under these stressful circumstances. Nurturing your relationship is just as important as achieving pregnancy. Taking a brief vacation from temperature charts, medication, or counting days will refresh you and enable you to try even longer. It's a great investment in time.

Just feeling tired may not be a compelling enough reason to take a break. After all, nobody expects this situation to be a picnic. Only you know how much pressure you can withstand. How will you know when it's time to take a breather? To some extent, it's an arbitrary choice. You just do it. One of you may feel more strongly about it than the other, but it's important for you both to express your feelings. One of you may feel the need to back off for a short time, and that may be the only signal you'll receive. Don't panic. Your need for a rest isn't an expression of disloyalty or a sign of weakness. The ability to recognize that it's time for a break is a very healthy thing.

Apart from your feelings, perhaps one of you is facing a particularly stressful time at work. Maybe you're going to have a houseful of relatives for the holidays. Or, you might open the newspaper and read about a now-or-never travel bargain. Factoring out infertility temporarily makes these situations easier to handle.

Don't be afraid that once you stop you won't get started again. If you have the motivation, it will not disappear because you wanted a vacation. On the contrary, you'll gain renewed energy. If you do find yourselves reluctant to begin again, that in itself is a signal worth exploring, and it was not caused by your break. Remember, it's natural to feel a need to rest and recuperate. Don't feel guilty about it. It's great sanity insurance for the future. Try it.

Distract Yourselves

Even if you can't find a way to take a break, there are ways you can give yourselves mental and physical distraction from the omnipresence of infertility.

If trying to have a baby is the only focus of your life right now, you risk burning yourselves out. You must try to make room in your lives for other things. It could be a hobby, a volunteer project, learning something new, or taking up a sport.

Try to enhance whatever interest you find by becoming something of an expert. Reading about a hobby can bring a sense of satisfaction and mastery that might be missing from other parts of your life. It will give you something new to talk about together and with others. If your new interest endures, you will have something to enrich yourselves for the rest of your life.

Being told to take up a hobby is to some extent useless; you can't force yourself to be suddenly interested in something new. A spark inside will tell you what you might like. Infertility's woes may have dampened your curiosity lately, so you should make an effort to find new things to get excited about. Once you open yourself up to these experiences it will get easier and easier. But at first, go ahead and push yourself. Look over this list and see what might appeal to you:

- **Theater: Attend performances** regularly, read the classics, follow the news of Broadway. Joining a local amateur troupe could really keep you busy!

- **Film: Videotaped classics** are now available everywhere. You can design your own film history course, study the work of certain actors or directors. Become an expert on westerns, detective films, screwball comedies. It's a great escape.

- **Opera: Regional companies** make this lively art available to more people than ever. Start with perennial opera favorites by Puccini or Verdi. Read a summary of the story, listen to the music at home first. Go to the theater and cry at the sad endings. Opera can be a great emotional release.

- **Sports: Take up** a sport you can enjoy together and separately, such as tennis. Physical activity is a *terrific* tension reliever. You may have to push yourself at first, but as you reach a stage of proficiency your enthusiasm will carry you along. If you'd like to go it alone, try jogging, aerobics, swimming. Try biking, hiking, even golf. Small talk with new sports buddies gives you a chance to chat about something other than your problems and provides a sense of fellowship.

- **Music: Tear yourselves** away from your familiar favorites, and explore a form of music new to you both. Jazz, new age, classical, postmodern, blues, and Broadway show tunes all offer rich opportunities for listening. Try a short music appreciation course; you may find certain types of music to be soothing and comforting.

- **Volunteer Work: Working** in the community to help those less fortunate can be satisfying and help bring perspective to your own life. You could tutor illiterate adults, coach a team on the weekends, feed the hungry, visit the sick, clean up the local park. Don't use volunteer work as a penance to buy worthiness, however. Choose a task you can stick with, and realize that doing good must be for its own sake.
- **Nature Studies:** A special attachment to nature can often develop as you try to start your family. As a hobby, you can fine-tune a love of nature through bird-watching, hiking, stargazing, rock-hunting, camping, identifying plants. You may want to involve yourselves in preservation or conservation work, too.
- **Gardening: Through houseplants,** in the backyard, or in a community plot, nurturing plants can be very satisfying. Flowers give wonderful natural beauty, and the physical labor can relieve tension. Homegrown vegetables taste better, too. Watching your plants grow provides a way to express loving and caring feelings.
- **Tinkering at Home:** Whether you live in an apartment or in a house, isn't there always something else to be done? Learn a skill you usually hire someone else to do for you. Even changing the washer on your faucet is a start. You'll have a new feeling of accomplishment.

Obviously, there are many other interests that you can investigate. If you pour a little of your energy into a chosen activity at least once a week, you may develop a pleasant routine that you can regularly look forward to. Even if your new hobby doesn't stick with you for life, you can still have the satisfaction of trying new things, and you will have something other than infertility to think and talk about.

Support Groups

If nobody around you seems to understand what you're going through, or if you need a place to speak more frankly about infertility, the atmosphere of a support group could be helpful to you. Getting together with several other couples and listening to one another can be an enormous relief. You can be completely yourself in a support group; there's no need to pretend that everything's fine when it isn't. You'll be with people who not only sympathize, but empathize with you. Support-group meetings can provide a refuge from the "fertile world" for an hour or two each week, and it's a place where you can learn about coping techniques, hear the stories of others' experiences, or simply unwind. Real work can go on in support groups, too. Couples like yourselves will help you gain perspective on your situation, and work along with you as you strengthen and move toward resolution.

Support groups are usually led by a professional who may be a social worker, a psychologist, or a counselor with experience in infertility. The leader brings structure to your meetings and helps maximize the benefit everyone can gain from attending.

Support groups can be found through many infertility specialists. Yours may be one of them, so be sure to ask. One of the basic services of most RESOLVE local chapters is to organize support groups for its members. In large cities, there are specialized support groups that can focus on a particular aspect of infertility. You will be given the name of a support-group leader who will talk with you and determine what type of group is most appropriate. There are fees that are paid to the group leader, but they are usually very reasonable.

Support groups meet for a defined period of time, usually between eight and twelve weeks. It is desirable to have an endpoint in sight as you meet weekly and talk, so that you have a sense of purpose, a goal of moving toward resolution. In the group you may develop intense, quickly forged friendships that sometimes carry over into other parts of your life. Whether you make friends with fellow members of the group or not, you will meet together and help each other in a unique way that you can feel proud of.

When Counseling Could Help

Infertility is a complex problem, both medically and emotionally. It may be one of the most complicated ones you'll have in your life. Couples often find that this is the first major setback in their relationship, and they might not have learned the dual coping skills to handle it yet. The emotional mine field of hope, despair, loss, grief, regret, anger, and bewilderment replaces a settled domestic life. Pulling together to give mutual support isn't always possible, and you might begin to feel the strain.

Some infertility specialists automatically recommend that couples see an infertility counselor at least once. Even if your doctor has never mentioned counseling to you, you could be wondering if it might help you. Here are some situations when couples find counseling beneficial:

- If marital problems caused by or aggravated by infertility persist or become overwhelming to one or both of you
- When you need to make a major decision regarding your treatment, and want to fully consider all medical and emotional aspects
- If you need experienced guidance to discuss together the intense stress you are feeling
- If you need more support than you are receiving from friends, family, a support group, or even one another
- If you don't really know what your goals are or why you are pursuing the goals you have now
- If you are considering stopping treatment altogether, and need help to think it through
- If you are trapped in one stage of treatment, and cannot make a decision to try an alternative
- If your behavior is changing adversely because of infertility and you are becoming concerned
- If your doctor won't or can't address the emotional difficulties that infertility causes, and you need a professional perspective
- If your sexual relationship is so out of kilter that you fear it won't recover after you've resolved your infertility
- If you feel uncontrollable despair, depression, panic, anger, or fear and need help understanding your feelings

You can find qualified infertility counseling through RESOLVE or through your specialist. Speaking to a prospective therapist on the telephone offers you a chance to ask about experience and qualifications, and it helps you get a "feel" for the person. If you can, try to indicate what sort of help you are looking for. Listen for a compassionate response.

Facing your first appointment can be frightening. A qualified professional will know that you are feeling nervous and will help you. You should be prepared to speak frankly. There are no wrong feelings, no bad answers. This is not the place to sugarcoat your feelings, gloss over adversity, ignore anger. Your therapist will help you to become more self-aware as well as better able to recognize the needs of your partner. You will learn about why you are feeling the way you do, why you're reacting to infertility the way you are. Contrary to discovering that you're out of control, going to a therapist a few times means that you're helping yourself—and that's healthy and good.

Commonly Prescribed Treatments for Women: What to Expect

Treatments for Ovulation Problems

Clomiphene Citrate (Clomid, Serophene) Clomid is one of the most common fertility drugs. Your doctor may prescribe it for you if you do not ovulate or have periods, if your ovulation is unpredictable, or if your periods are erratic. It may be given to you to help regulate luteal phase defect, or for polycystic ovarian disease. Be sure you understand your diagnosis, and why your doctor feels Clomid can help you.

Clomid is the safest of the "superdrugs." There are fewer side effects and those that do appear are less serious. It's effective, too: it will stimulate ovulation for about 75 percent of patients, and pregnancies occur in 65 percent of women for whom all other factors are normal.

Clomid therapy begins after your ovulation problems are well understood. You may have blood work or a vaginal smear to detect estrogen levels. You may have a shot of the hormone progesterone to induce your period. Most women start Clomid with a 50 milligram tablet taken on Day 3, 4, or 5 of the menstrual cycle. It is continued for five days. You will probably be told to monitor your basal body temperature.

Clomid does have some side effects. The usefulness of the drug outweighs the risk, but you should be carefully monitored nonetheless. Each month you should be checked by your doctor to be sure your ovaries have not been overstimulated. This checkup usually consists of a bimanual exam, which isn't painful. At home, watch for moodiness, sleep disturbances, hot flashes, fatigue, breast tenderness, nausea, and blurred vision. If you experience abdominal discomfort, pressure, or pain, call your doctor right away. In some cases, cervical mucus can be reduced by Clomid, and estrogen supplements will be prescribed.

Ask your doctor how long to expect to take Clomid, and keep a treatment plan for the future in mind. Most women take it for at least six months or so. If you have not responded within a reasonable time, you may be asked to consider taking a stronger fertility drug.

If Clomid helps you conceive, your odds of multiple births are not high. In fact, there is only a 5 to 10 percent chance for twins. The publicity surrounding most multiple births is usually associated with stronger drugs. The risk of miscarrying is 20 percent, the same as for any normal pregnancy.

Be sure to speak up to your doctor if you have any questions about taking Clomid. You can also contact RESOLVE for literature about this drug. Some women do have a hard time on Clomid, but for the majority of patients, this medication brings much-wanted results with a minimum of side effects. Bad experiences seem to result from an inadequate understanding of Clomid use by doctors, failure to carefully monitor for effects, or poor communication between doctor and patient. Keep a good relationship open with your specialist and you will do well.

Be Aware, Don't Be Scared

PAT KUNKEL

Once my doctor prescribed Clomid, I had such expectations and was so excited. Other than the possibility of ovarian cysts, no other side effects were discussed. My doctor stressed that monthly examinations for this possibility were a must. Other than this, all that concerned me was how our small house was going to accommodate twins!

Initially, I was on 50 milligrams a day, which is the lowest dosage. I really had no problems. Oh, there were hot flashes, but these were very mild and fairly infrequent. After reassurance from my doctor that these were common side effects, I did not worry. I felt that they were a small price to pay compared to the examinations and tests I had undergone during my husband's and my four-and-a-half-year struggle with infertility.

After some months passed with no success, the Clomid dosage was increased to 100 milligrams a day. Two days after this change, things began to happen. I typically read before retiring at night. This night, however, I found I was having great difficulty. Words and letters were swimming all over the pages. I rubbed my eyes, adjusted the intensity of my bedside lamp, but nothing seemed to help. Thinking I was tired, I shut off the light and went to sleep.

Other changes became evident. I became withdrawn, moody, and depressed. I no longer felt in control of myself. Again I called my doctor, this time in tears. My doctor sympathized with my depression and suggested I see a psychiatrist. "Many couples need help coping with the stress," he said. My head was swimming when I heard this. I asked if it could possibly be the medication. The doctor was adamant: no, it could not be the Clomid that was affecting me in this manner. I thought the situation was even more hopeless. Was I really crazy?

I called in a refill for my Clomid prescription. The pharmacist is an acquaintance of mine, who, I'd heard, had also taken Clomid. I mentioned the symptoms I was having. She did not sound surprised at all, and reported that the three years she was on Clomid are referred to as "that crazy time" by her and her husband. She then read the documented side effects to me. Everything

I had been experiencing was there in black and white! She saved the product insert for me.

One cannot imagine the relief both my husband and I felt! We went back to the doctor, and only then did he concede that my symptoms might be from the Clomid. Needless to say, I changed doctors!

I've learned that it is imperative that a physician listen to reactions that his individual patients are experiencing. Every patient is different. If your doctor does not know the answer, he must find out.

In the end, Clomid did help even out my monthly cycles. From now on, though, I am making sure my doctors explain all of the possible side effects to me!

Human Menopausal Gonadotropin (Pergonal) HMG, or Pergonal, is the fertility drug that you read about in the newspapers. It has the "miracle" qualities that give couples hope when they had none before. It is often associated with in vitro fertilization and a related technique called GIFT, which are both in the news and which will be discussed later.

Using Pergonal is a big step. It requires a commitment of emotional energy, physical strength, money, and time. Deciding for Pergonal therapy should be no snap judgment, no matter how anxious you are to become pregnant.

Knowing if this drug is right for you is crucial. Your doctor will explain to you why you might benefit. As you talk about Pergonal, make sure you know about your doctor's personal experience in administering and monitoring it, and ask about the odds of success.

How can you tell if you're ready yourself? Talk to not only your specialist, but also to members of the staff, who may see things the doctor doesn't. Find a contact person to speak with who has personal experience of Pergonal therapy. A fellow patient at your doctor's or a member of RESOLVE can help you. Talk to your partner; he will be very involved also, whether he likes it or not! Consider the costs of the drug itself, plus the expense of careful monitoring. Pergonal therapy is terribly expensive, often around $1,000 per cycle.

Pergonal is given by injection. Women can make repeated visits to the doctor's office for shots, but many elect to have them at home, administered by their partners. You will feel like a pincushion after a while, and the site of injections can become sore.

Monitoring is thorough and time-consuming. There are absolutely no shortcuts allowed. You will have daily ultrasound observation of your ovaries, to see how egg follicles are developing and to make sure your ovaries aren't overstimulated. Traditional ultrasound requires keeping the bladder full, so you could be uncomfortable, but it's completely painless. Blood work is also done on a daily basis.

Going to the doctor's so often could put your job into temporary limbo. Ask your doctor for a realistic assessment of how much time you must commit day by day, each month. Factor in waiting-room time. If working hours will be seriously threatened, consider taking sick days, moving up some vacation time, even changing working hours. Some women may take a leave of absence. Only you can figure out how you can best juggle your many commitments. Try to be realistic and give yourself every break you can.

Pergonal therapy usually starts on Day 3, 4, or 5 of your cycle. You will be tested for estrogen to see if the dosage is correct, and it could be adjusted after you begin. You will be monitored with pelvic exams and ultrasound. You may receive a shot of HCG (human chorionic gonadotropin) toward the middle of your cycle, which should stimulate ovulation to occur. During monitoring, if it is seen that you are developing too many follicles or the follicles are developing too rapidly, you will not be given this stimulation, and your ovaries will be left alone to rest.

If you are scheduled for the HCG shot, you'll probably be told to have intercourse twenty-four hours or so before ovulation, so sperm will be in your tubes as the eggs are released.

If no pregnancy results, your dosage may be adjusted for the next try. For some reason, the second month on Pergonal has better pregnancy odds. Ask your doctor. This regimen is tough, so you may not be encouraged to continue after four cycles. It is up to you to decide.

Be clear on how to monitor yourself for signs of ovarian hyperstimulation, which is the major risk of Pergonal therapy. If it occurs, it is usually mild, but in a few cases it can become severe. Watch for abdominal pain, swelling, pressure. If you experience any unusual sensation in your abdomen, have it checked without delay. Bed rest is often all that is required to recover from mild hyperstimulation.

Pergonal successfully induces ovulation in 90 percent of women. By two to four cycles, there is a 60 percent chance of pregnancy. These are amazing statistics for women who could not ovulate before. Multiple births do occur, but only in about 20 percent of cases. Most are twins. Triplets, quads, and quints are rare, and if you are being carefully watched, you and your doctor will know if you are developing multiple follicles. You can then elect to withhold your HCG shot. Be sure you and your doctor understand each other if this situation arises.

The highs and lows of infertility are already well known to you. Pergonal treatments can intensify these feelings. It offers the sweetest reward—pregnancy at last. This is a terrific motivator. But should one or two cycles pass before success, getting your period can be even more saddening. Keep your eyes open for these strong emotions and support each other as best you can. Enjoy the unique hope that this treatment can bring to you, and congratulate yourselves on your stamina—you've earned it.

I Just Needed a Little Help

ALICE DUNN

*T*he end of the year marked the end of my infertility workup; hysterosalpingogram, two postcoital exams, two endometrial biopsies, semen analyses, blood tests, and a laparoscopy and D & C. Diagnosis: mild endometriosis and high prolactin.

I took Parlodel to control my prolactin level, but still no pregnancy. Later, a second blood test indicated low progesterone. My doctor said this meant I wasn't ovulating well, and prescribed clomiphene citrate to regulate and improve the quality of ovulation. After four months, my temperature charts were still baffling, and the doctor announced he would put me on Pergonal the following month.

I was in shock. Pergonal was a powerful drug reserved for women who really had problems. I ovulated every month; I just needed a little help. Not Pergonal!

And wasn't this my last hope? There is really nothing beyond Pergonal besides in vitro fertilization? And how many women get pregnant that way?

I was scared and told my doctor. He explained that with Pergonal he has much more control over the situation because the drug works directly on the ovaries. He acknowledged that the treatment was anxiety-ridden but encouraged me to speak to him whenever I felt the need.

It took me a few days to adjust to all that had transpired, and then I awaited the arrival of my next period, signaling the start of my first cycle of Pergonal. I was actually excited when the bleeding came, a feeling I had long forgotten!

I made it through the first week of injections with little trouble. I would get a little anxious after each blood test, wondering whether my estrogen level was increasing. Each time I got a positive report it was a relief. The drug was working!

By Day 10 my doctor decided I would get the shot of HCG because he felt I was ready to ovulate. It was so exciting! My husband and I dutifully made love the next few nights and felt confident we'd "hit it."

A week later my progesterone level was tested and I debated with myself whether or not to call for the results. I held out until Day 22 and called. My level was four times what it had been in the past. A rush came over me and, naturally, I assumed I was pregnant. I tried so hard not to get my hopes up, but that's all I could think about. I imagined how I would tell my husband and dreamed about sharing this victory with my doctor.

Forty-eight hours later I felt the first twinge of cramps and saw spots of blood. But that didn't mean anything. I could still be pregnant with spotting and cramps, I told myself. I called the nurse in the office and began to cry on the phone.

When my third cycle of Pergonal still did not produce the long-awaited pregnancy, I had difficulty bouncing back from the disappointment. I decided to take a break from treatment. As I write this essay I am, for the first time in two and a half years, taking that break. I am taking a vacation from doctor's appointments, temperature charts, and timed sex, and it's something I recommend to anyone caught up in this monthly grind. A great burden has been lifted and I feel hopeful again. I plan to go back on Pergonal when I feel stronger. In the meantime, I am gradually remembering what life was like before infertility—and enjoying it!

Other Treatments For Ovulation Problems

Parlodel If your ovulation is abnormal due to elevated prolactin levels, you may be given the drug bromocriptine (brand name Parlodel). This is a safe drug, given in tablet form. It is taken several times per day on a full stomach. Your doctor will determine how long you should take it, but it could be either a very short time or indefinitely. Watch for nausea, headaches, or constipation, which are the commonly reported side effects. Your blood will be tested for prolactin while you are taking Parlodel. This drug does a good job in treating the microscopically small pituitary tumors that can cause elevated prolactin, so ask your doctor about this medication before other measures are taken.

GnRH A more recent development in ovulation stimulation is the use of a hormone pump which administers doses of the hormone GnRH (gonadotropin-releasing hormone) on a timed basis. This hormone alerts the pituitary to send signals to the ovaries. Because the ovaries are not being stimulated directly, GnRH is considered safer than Pergonal. With this method of treatment, a woman wears a tiny automatic pump the size of a cigarette pack, attached to a belt. This device feeds timed doses of GnRH into an IV, the needle of which is placed just under the skin. "The pump" is not widely used, and researchers are now working on GnRH synthetics that do not require it for timed dosage. Also, this therapy isn't yet available for most women who can benefit from it. If you live near a large city or a major research hospital, you may want to look for information on GnRH pumps. Only if this therapy is appropriate for you, and you are highly motivated to use it, would this be your answer. Keep in mind that it usually is not covered by insurance.

Treatment for Luteal Phase Defect

Problems with a woman's luteal phase, or the second half of the menstrual cycle, are pretty common. How serious they are depends on which doctor you ask. Some experts feel luteal phase defect (sometimes referred to as LPD) is blamed too often for infertility problems, while others feel it is grossly underestimated. Whatever your doctor thinks, be sure your initial workup is not interrupted just because a luteal phase defect has turned up. A complete picture of your reproductive health is still necessary.

During the luteal phase, the ruptured egg follicle on the ovary secretes progesterone, a hormone which helps prepare the endometrial lining and supports early pregnancy. Because a variety of factors have been identified as possible triggers of luteal phase defect, there is no set treatment. If your specialist has fully investigated your cycle with an endometrial biopsy and blood work, a theory will emerge, and you will be treated accordingly.

You may be given progesterone suppositories, which will supply this hormone that your body is not producing adequately. Treatment is begun after ovulation has occurred, with the suppositories administered every twelve hours. Only when your next period has begun should they be discontinued. You may have to have another endometrial biopsy to determine if this treatment is working. Be sure to find out how long to expect to stay on these suppositories, and exactly how they are used.

Clomid is sometimes given for luteal phase defect, if the cause is low estrogen or low levels of the hormone FSH. Oddly enough, some women already on Clomid for other reasons go on to develop luteal phase defect, so this presents a delicate balance! Watch your BBT chart carefully, and monitor your body signs for Clomid's side effects.

You may be told that a series of HCG shots will help make up for luteal phase inadequacy. The HCG can prolong the life of the ovary's corpus luteum, so that it will produce proper amounts of progesterone. Sometimes Clomid is combined with HCG. In rare cases, Pergonal may be combined with the HCG, but be careful. Ask why this is necessary, and be sure you understand the rigors of this treatment. You may want to get another opinion before undertaking this therapy.

If your sole diagnosis is luteal phase defect, try to obtain as much information as you can. RESOLVE can keep you up to date on how treatments can differ. Be sure all other factors in infertility have been checked in both of you. Consider asking for pain medication, and take it in advance for the endometrial biopsies—they are painful, but very quick. If you find after a long period of treatment that you are having too many of these procedures, speak up! Unfortunately, this test is the only sure way to read the lining of the uterus, but a compassionate physician will try to keep the number of biopsies to a minimum, or offer you some relief from the brief moment of pain. Luteal phase defect can be a difficult condition, but there are many solutions at hand.

Treatments for Endometriosis

Endometriosis is a fairly common condition, found in women between the ages of twenty-five and forty. Endometrial cells, which normally are located in the uterus only, can migrate to areas outside the uterus, swelling and bleeding as if in the womb. This causes scarring, which may impair fertility. Sometimes there are obvious clues to endometriosis, so be thorough when going over your medical history with your doctor. In many women there is no sign of this condition except for infertility.

Endometriosis can only be confirmed by visualization of the abdominal cavity during a diagnostic laparoscopy, a test which usually comes fairly late in a woman's workup. If your doctor has reason to suspect endometriosis, you may be asked to have a laparoscopy before other major tests.

Describing the severity of a case of endometriosis and ordering appropriate treatment for it is somewhat subjective. Doctors of the American Fertility Society have set down a classification system to examine and describe endometriosis, and to record the extent of damage. After your laparoscopy, ask for a rundown of what your doctor has found. During your laparoscopy, though theoretically a diagnostic procedure, minor to moderate cases of endometriosis can often be corrected with laser or other surgical techniques. Therefore, it's a good idea to know in advance what your doctor is planning to do if endometriosis is indeed found.

If you have endometriosis, contact the Endometriosis Association (PO Box 92187, Milwaukee, Wisconsin 53202) for literature and information. Coping with the stress of the condition and its treatment can be trying, so arm yourself with knowledge. You can get information through RESOLVE, too.

Questions About your Treatment for Endometriosis   The chances of being helped by medication or corrective surgery are very good. When you talk over your treatment with your doctor, you might consider the following questions:

- How severe is my case?
- How are cases similar to mine typically treated?
- What are the chances of success with this treatment?
- When can we start trying to conceive?
- How will you know if the treatment is working?
- If my case is mild, should we wait and see for a few months before using medication?

- Does my age present a factor of urgency? If so, does this change how I will be treated?
- If medication is prescribed, what is it? What are its side effects? Do the benefits outweigh these effects?
- Is this medication costly? Is it covered by insurance?
- If you recommend more surgery, why? Can we avoid it? What are the odds of success (pregnancy) as opposed to the threat of additional scarring?
- Can you keep my surgery minor, thus avoiding major abdominal work?
- If I have severe pain due to endometriosis, do you propose severing the appropriate nerve during surgery? Will this affect my bowel or bladder function? Would this affect labor if I become pregnant? Could medication for endometriosis help the pain instead?
- How will my response to medication or the results of surgery be checked?
- What are my risks of ectopic pregnancy?
- Should we consider in vitro fertilization as a possible alternative? What are the odds of in vitro fertilization success as balanced against corrective surgery?

Danazol (Danocrine) Danazol is a synthetic androgen (a male hormone) that is often prescribed for endometriosis. It has the effect of simulating menopause, which causes endometrial implants to cease their cycle of swelling and bleeding. It also promotes reduction of the implants. While this isn't a cure for endometriosis, it can improve your condition enough to allow you to become pregnant.

Danazol is used most often in mild cases of endometriosis, where it's usually the sole treatment. It can also be used for a few months prior to surgical removal of implants and repair of endometriosis-damaged ovaries or tubes.

Taken in tablet form, your dosage level will depend on the severity of your case and your body weight, among other factors. You'll probably start with 400-800 milligrams per day, taken in several doses. Doctors try to keep the dosage as low as possible to reduce side effects, but it may have to be adjusted upward if your estrogen level doesn't drop as expected or you have breakthrough bleeding. Expect to take danazol for around six months or so, during which your periods will cease and you won't be able to try to get pregnant. Ovulation usually returns four to six weeks after you stop the drug, and you'll have your best chances of conception for the following year or so.

No discussion of danazol you have with your doctor is complete without a clear explanation of what possible side effects come with this medication. Severe side effects are uncommon, but most women have experienced a mild version of one or two reactions. Most side effects subside when you discontinue the drug, but alas, not all.

Danazol is a synthetic male hormone designed to help shut down the female hormones that aggravate endometriosis. While it helps control endometriosis it may also cause oily skin, acne, weight gain, hot flashes, mood swings, increased perspiration, muscle cramps, changes in appetite, an increase in body hair, and growth or darkening of facial hair. If you develop severe headaches, feel very depressed, or experience other serious changes, notify your doctor immediately.

If you are concerned about weight gain, you should know that weight gained from danazol may not be as simple to lose as weight gained from other medications. The gain is caused by a change in body proteins, and you're gaining muscle, not water weight. Talk over this fact with your doctor, and decide how you will handle this.

This sounds like an awesome list, but remember that the incidence of these effects is usually mild, and no woman gets them all. Some doctors may wish to brush aside your questions about side effects, but you have a right to know what to expect just in case.

GnRH Analogue Treatment with a synthetic form of GnRH is being developed and used in some major medical centers. This medication will shrink endometrial implants, and is an alternative to danazol that many women find they much prefer. It may be taken as a nasal spray. See if this medication is appropriate or available for you. It may be very expensive and may not be covered by most insurance plans, so make your medication decision carefully.

Corrective Surgery for Endometriosis Severe cases of endometriosis that do not respond to medication alone may require more surgery. After your diagnostic laparoscopy, your doctor will have a plan of attack, which could involve another laparoscopy or major abdominal surgery, called a laparotomy.

For a few months before surgery, you may be given medication such as Lupran or Danocrine to shrink swelling of endometrial implants, and facilitate their removal. Some doctors advocate following surgery with more medication, and some feel patients should go ahead and begin trying to conceive. Ask about the severity of your case, and how soon you can start trying again. If you're afraid that you are up against the clock, make these feelings known.

Who will be your surgeon? Find out if your prospective surgeon will use laser techniques to vaporize implants, if they will be cauterized (burned), or if they will be snipped and removed. Doctors and patients are excited about the results of laser surgery, because it often reduces bleeding and scarring, so ask about it for your case. It requires skilled and experienced hands, however.

A very severe case of endometriosis may call for full abdominal surgery, the laparotomy. Instead of a Band-Aid-sized puncture for laparoscopy, the laparotomy involves opening up the abdomen, a week in the hospital, and extended recovery time at home. This is a serious step, and you should take time to think about it and work out if this is right for you. Obtain a second opinion, as patients should always do for any proposed major surgery.

If you will have a laparotomy, ask about what corrections are to be made, and the surgical techniques that will be used. Can lasers be used? Ask about the extra care that will be taken to reduce scarring, bleeding, or additional formation of adhesions. Ask if your odds of pregnancy with in vitro fertilization techniques might match those with corrective laparotomy. Find out how long you will be under general anesthesia, in the hospital, off the job. You must factor in lost income as well as all costs. Try to be as well prepared financially, emotionally, and support-wise as you must be physically for this surgery.

Have you been told that your endometriosis is so severe, your pain so intense, that a hysterectomy is needed? Even if you yourself are begging for pain relief, please get at least one other opinion. You should not have to part with your uterus or ovaries until many other avenues of help are tried. Keeping your organs intact while treating your endometriosis should be your doctor's highest priority.

Treatments for Fallopian Tubes

The fallopian tubes perform several vital functions in reproduction, yet they are so delicate and vulnerable to damage! Endometriosis, pelvic inflammatory disease, sexually transmitted disease, infections, and adhesions from previous surgery have all been identified as culprits in harming the tubes. Often damage can occur quickly and without a woman's knowledge. Sometimes a severe infection followed by inflammation is noticed, but not caught in time. IUD-related infections have also been blamed.

Fallopian tubes are blocked or deformed by these problems. Medication can clear up an infection, but there is no pill to fix a physically damaged tube. Surgical repair is the only method. Fortunately, specialists are always working on improved techniques of tubal repair, and progress is being made.

Tubal problems will probably show up on the hysterosalpingogram. If more investigation is necessary, the laparoscopy allows examination of the outer tubes, and in a few cases, a doctor will look directly inside the tubes with a viewing scope. Your condition will be spelled out, and repairs that give the best odds of succeeding will be considered. Ask all the appropriate questions as you discuss your surgery (see the general questions under "Questions to Ask If You Need Surgery").

Surgeons are increasingly trying to avoid the laparotomy, which opens up the abdomen, but it's often a necessity for tubal repair. Ask if there's a chance for corrections to be made with a laparoscopy. With well-trained surgeons, several instruments can be used simultaneously to make repairs without laparotomy. Avoiding major surgery whenever possible is always an objective.

When considering your laparotomy for tubal repair, ask about the use of microsurgical techniques, which keep physical trauma to a minimum. Surgeons now make every effort to reduce extra damage that can be caused by the procedure itself. In microsurgery the surgeon cuts, sews, and repairs tissue on a very small scale, leaving more of the surrounding tissue unharmed than with traditional surgical techniques. The use of lasers to vaporize tissue that was once removed by cutting will often reduce the amount of bleeding. Special techniques keep the abdominal organs moist so that recovery time can be reduced. Incisions are made as small as possible.

As you talk with your doctor or surgeon about these issues, be sure to ask about training and experience in these procedures. Ask about the success odds you will have. Compare these odds with your odds if you elect to try in vitro fertilization instead. (Compare costs, too!) How complex is your tubal damage, and how well can it be repaired? What are the risks of subsequent ectopic pregnancy? How can you be watched for ectopic pregnancy? Because there are no guarantees of success with any one method, you must weigh all possibilities before you make your decision.

Help for Uterine Problems

Clues to uterine abnormalities may initially turn up in your medical history. Physical evidence of a problem might be found during your initial physical and pelvic exam, and confirmed by hysterosalpingogram. When your doctor is hot on the trail of a uterine problem, you may have a hysteroscopy, which is similar to the laparoscopy. A viewing scope will be inserted through the uterine wall or cervix to look directly inside for adhesions, scarring, fibroids, or inner shape abnormalities. Some of this damage results from previous surgery, inflammation from IUD use, or infection from sexually transmitted diseases. Abnormalities of shape can result if your mother took the drug DES while pregnant with you.

Surgical correction by hysteroscopy can often remove adhesions, and doctors have devised a balloon-like device that will keep the walls of the uterus from sticking back together after your operation. Doctors want to avoid making a full incision on the uterus, as with a laparotomy, because doing so means you will need a Caesarean section delivery should you become pregnant. Uterine fibroids that are very minor are usually left alone, while a few moderate ones might be removed with laser surgical techniques during hysteroscopy. Be sure to check out how carefully your surgeon plans to avoid excess bleeding, scarring, or re-adhesion, all of which helps keep your pregnancy odds as high as possible.

In cases of severe developmental abnormalities, such as a thick septum (a wall of tissue dividing the uterus), you may need a laparotomy for surgical correction. The same holds true if your doctor feels you have large fibroids that must be removed (in an operation called a myomectomy) or very extensive scarring. Always get another opinion before you decide to schedule any major surgery.

Treatment of the Cervix and Cervical Mucus

Infertility related to the cervix is of two types. First, the physical structure of the cervix may be damaged from previous infection or surgery, or from developmental abnormalities. Second, the cervix may not be producing the best mucus to promote sperm transport towards the egg. Your physical examination will reveal most structural problems, while a postcoital test can turn up evidence of sperm and mucus interaction difficulties or infection, and can document poor mucus production.

Some of the physical abnormalities could be developmental, that is, present from birth. If your mother took the drug DES while she was pregnant with you, it may have affected your reproductive organs. DES-related problems include a tightly closed cervix that must be gradually dilated. You may have severe scarring on your cervix, which affects its physical properties as well as impairing its production of mucus. If you are a DES daughter, you need a thorough examination performed with this fact in mind. You should be wary of any estrogen therapy for cervical mucus problems, so ask your doctor what's best. Please see the subsection called "DES exposure."

A most difficult problem is identified in medical language as incompetent cervix. This unfortunate nomenclature refers to a cervix that is not strong enough to "hold in" a pregnancy all the way to term. It is tragic that this physical problem cannot be diagnosed until a woman miscarries repeatedly after twelve weeks of pregnancy. In cases of DES daughters, the threat of incompetent cervix is recognized, and women can be carefully watched. Portable monitors are being devised that can detect premature dilation. A weak cervix can be stitched to make it stronger through the late stages of pregnancy, and then the stitches are removed for labor to begin.

Inadequate production of mucus can have a hormonal cause, or it may be due to scarring or other cervical damage from previous surgery or from infection. If you have an estrogen deficiency, you may receive supplements of this hormone in tablet form. If you are taking Clomid for ovulation regulation or induction, it can have the side effect of reducing the quality of your mucus, and you could be given estrogen for this as well. Ask your doctor about the most recent thinking on the safety of estrogen therapy, especially if you are a DES daughter. Estrogen can have some side effects, including altering your regular cycle, and doses should be as low as possible.

The presence of infections, especially sexually transmitted diseases such as gonorrhea, chlamydia, or ureaplasma, can affect cervical mucus and make it a poor swimming medium for sperm. You could be producing antibodies against infection that will attack sperm as well. The mucus itself may become chemically inhospitable for sperm, even on the best days of your cycle. If your postcoital test has revealed abnormalities, having your mucus cultured for infections is important. In cases where infection is found, both partners must be tested if any therapy is to work properly. In addition, infection may spread up through the uterus and damage tubes if it is not caught quickly.

For infection, you both will probably be treated with antibiotics of the tetracycline family. They can make you queasy, and you should avoid becoming pregnant while on these drugs. You will need to be retested to see if the medication has succeeded in clearing up your infection, and another postcoital examination is essential.

Should your difficulties continue, bear in mind that you can bypass the mucus altogether with intrauterine artificial insemination of your partner's sperm, a procedure called IAIH for short. In some cases, in vitro fertilization or GIFT procedure may be recommended, which is a more complex way to bypass the mucus.

Treatment of Immunity Problems in the Couple

Immunity problems between partners can manifest themselves in the mucus, semen, or the blood serum of either partner. This problem can be traumatic, and patience is needed to see it through, but treatment can be successful.

With this problem, a woman may manufacture antibodies to attack the sperm cells of her partner alone, or the sperm of any man. In rare cases, a man may manufacture antibodies against his own sperm. Thorough but expensive cross-testing of sperm, mucus, and blood may be required. If you have this problem, consider going to an expert, such as an andrologist, to have these tests made. Call your local RESOLVE for names of andrologists and labs that can do this work. There is a lot of debate in the medical community about immunity problems in infertility, and you will want the latest information.

A simple if old-fashioned way to try and overcome a woman's immunity reaction is using condoms during intercourse for six months or so. Having no direct contact with semen may lessen the woman's immune response over time. When you resume unprotected intercourse, your immune systems may be caught by surprise, and the sperm will get through unscathed. Keep in mind that you should try this method **only** if you feel you have plenty of time to try, and only if you want to completely avoid medical intervention. It's probably a better idea to treat immunity problems directly.

Once the partner with the immune reaction is determined, a program of therapy with steroids could be prescribed. This regimen will lower your overall immunity, so talk about it carefully. The doses can be kept low, and you should be given them on a limited basis.

As with mucus problems, artificial insemination (IAIH) can be used in cases of immune reactions. The sperm is "washed," that is, processed to separate them from seminal fluid that may contain antibodies produced by the reaction. The processed sperm can then be placed directly into the uterus, bypassing the cervical mucus. In vitro fertilization or GIFT might interest you if this therapy method doesn't work after a reasonable number of attempts.

DES Exposure

Diethylstilbestrol (DES) is a synthetic estrogen that was prescribed for pregnant women in hopes of preventing miscarriage. From the late 1940s into the 1960s, children were born who were directly affected by DES.

It has become known that daughters of women given DES have a greater frequency of malformation of their reproductive organs and a higher incidence of infertility problems than the general population. In addition, they should be monitored for the development of abnormal cells in the vagina or cervix which could be precancerous. DES sons can be found to have small or undescended testicles, or cysts in the epididymis. Problems with poor sperm quality have been associated with DES sons as well.

If you were born during the DES years and you have infertility problems, it's important to stop and consider if this drug was given to your mother. You may be able to ask her directly, but in many cases DES children cannot. If you suspect DES is a factor in your infertility, you may have to do some investigating of your mother's medical records. Help is available from DES Action National, Long Island Jewish Hospital, New Hyde Park, New York 11040. This organization acts as an educational clearinghouse for DES-affected persons and can provide you with information on how to do the necessary search.

In the meantime, your doctor should give you a special examination with DES in mind. Some abnormalities will show up in a simple pelvic exam or through a hysterosalpingogram. However, DES women need a special, painless, pelvic exam with a device called a colposcope, which aids the doctor's search for abnormal or irregular cells in the vagina or at the cervix. Lab studies similar to a Pap smear are conducted to further test for DES problems.

Above all, if DES is a factor in your life, be sure all your doctors treating your infertility know it. DES daughters who become pregnant should be watched carefully for a weakened cervix or other problems. If you feel you need a doctor who is more knowledgeable about DES-related problems, contact DES Action National for a referral. Throughout your life you should stick with a doctor who understands DES cases, whether or not you are trying to become pregnant.

DES-Related Infertility

JEAN QUINN MANZO

*M*y mother was given a prescription drug when she was pregnant with me to prevent a threatened miscarriage. DES, marketed under approximately two hundred brand names, is causing infertility problems in both men and women twenty to forty years after the drug was prescribed for their mothers.

After a year of trying and no baby, I consulted a fertility specialist. He asked me to "ask my mother"—as every gynecologist should. As my mother did not remember receiving medication nor were her medical records available, I consulted a DES specialist who concurred with the first doctor's diagnosis.

I am a classic case: T-shaped uterus, extremely small; luteal phase defect; incompetent cervix. While 81 percent of DES daughters will have a successful pregnancy, I am not one of them. Advised that I would need drugs to become pregnant, drugs to maintain the pregnancy, a stitched cervix, months of bed rest, and I "might" make seven months, my husband and I decided adoption was for us.

Infertility is devastating to deal with but in my ignorance I associated DES exposure with cancer and believed I had been given a death sentence. The organization DES Action has been of enormous help to me. Learning the risk of cancer was minimal was a comfort.

Tell your doctor you are a DES daughter. If she doesn't think that is critical information, find another doctor. DES daughters need special examinations regularly, and must have their pregnancies closely monitored.

My husband and I adopted an infant boy from Korea, and two years later, adopted a second. It has been five years since all this happened and the pain of infertility has faded away. My DES exposure helped me put my infertility in perspective.

A Warning: Pelvic Inflammatory Disease

PID stands for pelvic inflammatory disease, which is characterized by inflammation inside the pelvic cavity. The inflammation can be caused by infections, especially caused by sexually transmitted diseases, which invade the uterus and tubes. It could also result from a ruptured appendix, or a problem with an IUD, as well as past surgeries or an injury to the pelvic cavity.

PID is very common. Nearly a million women have it, in varying levels of severity, each year. Because of the prevalence of sexually transmitted diseases, many of which go undetected, the complication of PID has become an epidemic.

As the pelvic cavity becomes inflamed from the fight against infection, the body fights back as best it can. The result is scar tissue that can damage the fallopian tubes, or smother the reproductive organs, inhibiting their function. Even in cases that do not seem severe, fertility can be threatened or lost.

Repair of the damage brought on by PID can be as simple as a few snips during laparoscopy to remove scar tissue, or as sad and complex as a laparotomy to take out your irreparably damaged tubes.

Going over your medical history carefully with your doctor could reveal a bout of "flu" that was actually PID. Try not to overlook any clues from the past. As for the present, avoiding sexually transmitted diseases as well as watching for any vaginal infection cannot be stressed enough. In a monogamous couple this may sound like a strange proviso, but there it is. If you develop any symptoms that could point to an infection, get appropriate medical attention immediately. This applies to you at any time, whether or not you are trying to become pregnant.

The Special Problem of Miscarriage

You could be reading this section for two different reasons. First, you may have had two or more spontaneous abortions (the correct medical term for miscarriage), and you or your doctor now feel you could have an infertility problem. Or, you have succeeded in becoming pregnant after battling infertility, and you are concerned about the possibility of miscarrying. Both are legitimate and understandable concerns.

If you have had two or more miscarriages in the early weeks of pregnancy, it is very possible that you are the unfortunate victim of random, blighted pregnancies. But after two to three miscarriages, it is time to try to prevent any more. If there is a reason this is happening, a reason that perhaps can be found through infertility investigation, consider looking for it. It may help to ease your anxiety for your future pregnancies. Talk to your obstetrician frankly about the value of a few well-chosen tests. You may be referred to a specialist or you can find one on your own.

If you have been miscarrying later in your pregnancies, it is all the more urgent to search out a reason. It is sad to note that many miscarriages just cannot be explained, but if a problem can be found it is well worth searching for.

Relieving your anxiety is also important if you are finally pregnant after infertility. Whether naturally conceived, or helped along by new technologies, your pregnancy is precious! Worry that you might lose it is natural. But you should realize that the great majority of women who become pregnant after infertility go on to have normal, healthy babies. The chances of miscarriage are indeed somewhat higher for women over thirty-five who have had infertility problems, but the odds are not so high that you must walk around on tiptoe. Far from it. Remember that if you had a good workup, your condition is well-known to your doctors, and many risks of miscarriage have already been completely eliminated. If you go over your workup one more time with your doctor, you'll be better able to enjoy your pregnancy.

Clues to Infertility-Related Miscarriage

Here are some factors in infertility-related miscarriage, and the tests of the workup that can reveal them:

Physical and Pelvic Exam, Medical History

- DES exposure
- occupational or environmental hazards, lifestyles that promote risk

Blood Work

- hormonal problems, such as prolactin or progesterone imbalances
- immune reaction (this is controversial as a cause of miscarriage)
- genetic problems, found in special karyotyping test

Cultures of Cervical Mucus

- chronic infections such as ureaplasma

Endometrial Biopsy

- luteal phase defect

Hysterosalpingogram

- uterine shape abnormalities
- risk of ectopic pregnancy due to damaged or deformed tubes
- fibroids or polyps
- Asherman's syndrome (walls of uterus adhere to one another)

Laparoscopy

- endometriosis: in mild cases, increased prostaglandins may be associated with muscle contractions. Endometriosis-damaged tubes could be the cause of ectopic pregnancies.

Watching for an Ectopic Pregnancy

If you are at increased risk of ectopic pregnancy due to endometriosis, PID, or tubal damage, you should be watched carefully in the very early days after you conceive. Your blood can be monitored for the proper rise in hormones, which will indicate that the pregnancy has implanted in the uterus. If the blood work shows an abnormality, you can be checked with ultrasound. Ask your doctor about the beta-HCG test while you are still trying to conceive, and you'll be reassured that you're well prepared.

Whenever you discuss the odds of miscarriage with your doctor, or read statistics connected with certain conditions, treatments, or drugs, do not panic. The baseline statistic of the incidence of all miscarriage is a full 20 percent in the normal, fertile population. That is, 20 percent of *all* pregnancies are lost. So, when you see that the miscarriage rate for Clomid is 20 percent, you now know that this is the same risk as for any pregnancy. This percentage is a fact of obstetrics, and while it may seem high, knowing this rate gives the miscarriage risks for post-infertility pregnancies valuable perspective.

If You Are Still Worried

The information about infertility-related causes of miscarriage you've just read may help you stop thinking, "But what if . . . ?" and allow you to put extraneous worries about miscarriage out of your mind. But if you are still wondering what might happen if you threaten to miscarry, or what you should do to facilitate finding the cause of a miscarriage, here is a list of points to go over with your doctor. You should seek every reassurance from your medical professionals and realize one important point: miscarriage is not a life-threatening event for the mother. It can be frightening, but you will recover, usually very quickly. The emotional impact of miscarriage is great, and you must mourn the loss. But friends, family, and health-care workers around you will support you, and gradually, over time, you will begin to feel better.

What to Do In Case of Miscarriage

Read together about what actions should be taken in the event of a miscarriage, and double-check them with your doctor's views:

1. Report any spotting to your doctor immediately. Spotting happens in many pregnancies and does not mean you are going to miscarry. Most spotting will go away and you will have a normal pregnancy. But do not take a chance. Call and report all details: when it began, how much, color. Carefully follow your doctor's instructions.

2. Keep in mind that if you do begin to miscarry, neither you nor your doctors can stop it or save the pregnancy. Medical intervention will be ordered when necessary to help you recover and heal from the miscarriage, but sadly, once a spontaneous abortion is underway, there's nothing your doctor can do.

3. If you begin to miscarry, try to get some support right away. After calling the doctor, call your partner, a friend, a relative, a neighbor. You do not have to handle this alone! Even if you don't need to go to the hospital, you will need emotional support. A second set of ears to help hear the doctor's instructions and help you follow them is invaluable.

4. Miscarriages are very different from one another, but there are no "easy" ones. If you are having a painful miscarriage with much

bleeding, your partner or a supportive friend or relative will help you deal with it. Here is what they can do for you:

a) If possible, the passed products of conception should be collected for examination. This may yield valuable information about the cause of this miscarriage.

b) Make the woman as comfortable as possible, help her change into clean clothes, change the sheets if necessary, give emotional as well as practical support. It is essential.

c) NO PLATITUDES! This is a crisis, and glib sayings on the nature of miscarriage are completely inappropriate.

d) Call the woman's doctor, put her on the phone, then have the doctor repeat instructions to you.

e) If hospitalization is necessary, arrange transportation and insist that the woman be placed in a room away from newly delivered mothers.

f) Be sure the woman's spouse has unlimited access to her room.

g) Please let the couple talk about the miscarriage as much as they need to, even if they want to recount graphic details. Don't give advice or draw conclusions, just listen.

h) Be sympathetic and understanding on the due date, even if it is many months in the future.

There are support groups available for couples who have experienced miscarriage, which can be very helpful. Call RESOLVE and speak to a contact person if you need one-on-one support. Give yourselves time to recover emotionally at your own natural pace. Don't chide yourselves to "buck up!" right away. After experiencing grief, life will begin to resemble normalcy, and you may wish to begin trying again. When you are ready to accept hearing it, it is encouraging to remember that most couples can go on to have a healthy baby, even after several miscarriages.

Miscarriage

Dorothy J. Hagerty

*M*iscarriage. It's an event that most people never talk about because they don't know what to say. At least that's the way it was for me. The statistics indicate that approximately 20 percent of all pregnancies end in miscarriage. Well, let me tell you, that doesn't make it any easier to deal with if it happens to you.

My miscarriage was diagnosed as a missed abortion at twelve and a half weeks, and a D & C was scheduled five days later. Our first reaction was one of disbelief. Surely the ultrasound was wrong, but it wasn't. For about ten days I was in emotional shock and I cried very little. My first day back to work was horrible because my emotional subconscious started to take down that protective barrier around me. One of the women I worked with was three weeks ahead of me in her pregnancy, and she was the last person I wanted to see. I cried uncontrollably that evening and thought for sure I was losing my mind. When I had a checkup the following day with my doctor, he took the time to talk with me about my emotional needs, and only then did I realize that I was going through the natural, beginning steps of grieving. Let me share my doctor's insight with you.

First, your body is changing hormonally (once again), and therefore some of your emotions are a direct result of that. Second, if you had a D & C, you are physically recovering from that as well. Third, you have just suffered a sudden and unexpected loss. You don't have to have something to touch in order to grieve. My baby was very real to me. I saw its heartbeat at eight weeks and I emotionally held that baby in my arms every night. Bonding for me, as for many infertile couples, came very early in my pregnancy. The loss of my baby was just as real to me as if it had been born, which is a very normal feeling to have.

When I was able to understand what I was going through emotionally, mentally, and physically, I was then able to move ahead and put my grief into perspective. Don't deny yourself the time and energy it takes to grieve. And remember that you will grieve differently than your spouse. Cry; get angry; scream; question God, yourself, and your doctors to bring grief to the surface so you can deal with it. I read as many books as possible on miscarriage and also found that writing about my loss, as I'm doing now, is very therapeutic. Do whatever you need to do to see yourself through this very difficult time. Confront it, find your own way to handle it, and you will get through, as difficult as it may seem now. You have a right to grieve, and there is no reason to be ashamed of your hurt.

Whatever you do, try not to let it destroy you. Our loss happened over seven months ago, and when the woman at work had her baby I was angry and resentful. When my own due date arrived, I hurt deeply inside. But I was able to deal with these emotions because I knew why they existed. Learn about your own feelings and you too will be able to see that ray of hope at the end of the tunnel.

Commonly Prescribed Treatments for Men: What to Expect

The Varicocele

A varicose vein in the testicle, or varicocele, is very commonly cited as a cause of male infertility. This enlarged vein will be found during a physical exam, but first clues to the problem will show up in the semen analysis. A low count, sometimes accompanied by poor motility, can be the result of the added heat that this condition causes in the scrotum.

Many men who have had no fertility problems have a varicocele. In fact, 15 percent of all men have this condition. But about 40 percent of infertile men show a varicocele, and its correction does offer a chance to increase the sperm count. However, be sure that your partner has been thoroughly checked and that any causes of female infertility are also being treated.

If you have time to wait, you don't have to rush right into surgery. Trying less invasive methods of scrotal cooling might help you. Even if they sound slightly frivolous, in some cases they work. The obvious first action is wearing looser-fitting undershorts, which will give your scrotum a chance to use its natural cooling tendencies. Think about your work situation. Are you exposed to heat, sitting all day? There are scrotal cooling devices available, resembling an athletic cup, which can be worn in order to keep the testes at the proper temperature. Ask your doctor about these possibilities. You'll have to wait at least three months to see if these methods may do any good, so have patience. You can always schedule surgery after trying these methods.

When you and your doctor agree it's time to tackle the varicocele, you need the services of a urologist who is also a surgeon. You will undoubtedly get a referral, but you will want to ask about experience, success rates, chances of the condition coming back, and the possibility of bilateral (both sides) correction. You will be admitted to the hospital and go under general anesthesia, although this is not considered a major surgical procedure.

The traditional method of correcting a varicocele is to surgically tie off the varicose scrotal vein. The surgeon makes a small incision to the left and a little above the pubic area (or on both sides for a bilateral), and the vein is found right below; there is no need to delve into the pelvic cavity. The vein is severed and tied off. The blood has other paths to use for travel, so this does not injure or impair you in any way. In skilled hands, this procedure is very quick, so you will not be under anesthesia for very long.

You will experience pain and discomfort in the abdomen for a period of one week to perhaps two weeks. You may have some swelling. Watch for infection at the incision site, and report any undue pain to your urologist. You can resume normal activities in about a week, and can be completely active in about two weeks. You will probably have to take two or three days off from your job, but after thorough rest over the weekend, you may be able to return to work the following week.

Before going in, be sure you understand what's going to happen, why it's recommended for you, what alternatives might exist, costs, insurance coverage, recovery timetable, complication risks. Your doctor can explain all these matters, but may not be able to fully explain why this operation works. It's not fully understood. However, most doctors feel the results, a higher sperm count in many cases, speak for themselves.

Also, you may want to ask about the "balloon" method of treating your varicocele. In this method, the vein is blocked not by tying it off, but by placing a tiny silicone balloon device inside the vein. The balloon is placed in the vein by an interventional radiologist. This specialist uses x-ray visualization to properly position the tiny balloon during an outpatient procedure. There is no incision, only a puncture where a catheter is introduced into the vein, and local anesthetic is issued. There is considerably less pain involved than with traditional surgery, and virtually instantaneous recovery time.

As great as it sounds, the balloon method has its drawbacks. It is not yet widely performed, there is the risk of x-ray exposure, and there is a chance that the balloon may "travel" to another location through the vein. Find out all you can.

After your varicocele has been corrected, you have the long wait of three months or more to see if your sperm count improves. These first months after the procedure can be trying. If your count has not risen satisfactorily, a regimen of Clomid therapy (yes, the same drug given to women) or a program of HCG injections may help. There is no guarantee that either treatment will work, but in some cases these medications can support the sperm manufacturing process and help your count go up. There are side effects to the HCG shots, and the term of treatment can be longer than you'd like, so be thoughtful as you talk about this additional treatment. You and your doctor may want to use your somewhat improved count as basis for a program of artificial insemination, or perhaps for in vitro fertilization or GIFT. Don't forget to consider all the alternatives appropriate to your case.

Treatments for Male Hormonal Problems

Hormonal imbalances are found far less often in men than in women, but they can cause poor sperm counts in about 20 to 25 percent of infertile men. If your count is low enough to be a concern and there is no varicocele, you will probably have blood work to determine your hormone levels.

If your infertility seems to be due to a hormonal problem, are you seeing a specialist who is experienced in diagnosing and treating these conditions? A urologist or andrologist may be better able to interpret your blood work and decide what medication you need. Ask your present infertility specialist how many cases similar to yours have been treated in the past, and with what success. Be sure this diagnosis is based on more than one semen analysis, and that your medical history and current lifestyle have been studied for clues to a lowered sperm count.

Until recently, men were often told their counts were poor due to a thyroid problem. This is now known to be a rare cause of infertility in men. Additionally, a thyroid problem would manifest itself in other ways apart from an abnormal semen analysis. Don't let a doctor treat you for a thyroid condition unless it is demonstrable by other symptoms and is confirmed by blood work.

Clomiphene Citrate (Clomid, Serophene) For low counts and/or poor motility, doctors sometimes prescribe Clomid, which acts on the male hormonal system as well as the female's. In men, it can be given to help several different conditions, so go over your precise diagnosis with your specialist and learn what Clomid may be able to do for you. In men, the treatment regimen usually consists of taking a low dose of Clomid (administered in tablet form) daily for twenty-five days, skipping five days, then taking it again for twenty-five more days. Blood work will show if the drug is having any effect. There are some side effects to Clomid, so be aware of blurry vision or breast tenderness. An increased sex drive is possible. There is a very small chance of liver damage, so if this is a concern, ask your doctor how your liver function can be monitored. Overall, risk and side effects of Clomid are very minor.

Human Chorionic Gonadotropin (HCG) If your specialist wants to stimulate your testicles to produce testosterone and start or increase sperm production, a program of HCG injections may be recommended to you. In some cases, HCG will be supplemented with Pergonal (human menopausal gonadotropin). Ask what specific benefit this should bring, and get an estimate of your odds of increasing your count. Proceed carefully, since this therapy can be inconvenient, uncomfortable, and expensive. The injections are needed several times a week for some time, and the medication can alter your sex drive. Doctors disagree on the value of this therapy, but if it is your only chance, you may want to give it a try. You might be able to bring your count up to normal, or perhaps up far enough for artificial insemination techniques to be viable.

Bromocriptine (Parlodel) Men as well as women may have elevated prolactin levels, which could interfere with fertility. In some cases, high prolactin can affect potency. Hyperprolactinemia is treated in men with the same drug as in women—bromocriptine. Taking Parlodel (the brand name of bromocriptine tablets) is simple and has few or no side effects.

If you are diagnosed with hyperprolactinemia, has your doctor ruled out a pituitary tumor as the cause? If there is reason to suspect one of these noncancerous, microscopic-sized tumors, you may be asked to have a CAT-scan, which is a noninvasive x-ray of the skull. It is completely painless. Your doctor will guide you on to further treatment if it is necessary, but all you may need is a treatment program with Parlodel.

Other Therapies Cortisone therapy is sometimes used in connection with disorders of the adrenal gland. If this is your problem, proceed carefully, and ask about dosage levels, side effects, and the odds of elevating your sperm count. Some doctors do not feel this therapy is very effective, while others do, so you may want to get a second opinion.

Testosterone is given to restore male characteristics that never developed or have diminished due to testicular damage from illness or infection. This may or may not affect your sperm count, even if the male characteristics do respond. In other cases, doctors have administered testosterone to "jump start" the testicles to produce sperm, but this rebound often does not occur. You and your doctor must decide if it is worth trying, and your information will be more complete with another medical opinion, preferably from an andrologist.

Blockage of Sperm Ducts: Surgical Repair

Microsurgical techniques have made the delicate repair of sperm ducts possible in many cases of vasectomy reversal and of blockages due to infection or developmental abnormality. Your doctor may suspect a blockage after interpreting your semen analysis and/or ruling out varicocele and hormone imbalances. To confirm and pinpoint this diagnosis, you will probably have to have a testicular x-ray, or vasogram. Since this test is performed under general anesthesia, you may have it in conjunction with your surgical repair. Ask if you can save yourself this extra dose of general anesthetic in this way.

Many blockages due to infection are caused by sexually transmitted diseases such as ureaplasma or chlamydia. These diseases often show no symptoms and aren't discovered until infertility is diagnosed. Sometimes previous surgery performed near the ducts, such as a hernia repair, can accidentally sever ducts. In vasectomy, the ducts are severed intentionally.

If you are a candidate for surgery of this type, choose your surgeon carefully. Ask for a doctor experienced and skilled in microsurgery, and find out the general odds of success in cases of your type. These procedures require steady, patient hands, and you want a surgeon who has a high rate of success. Call RESOLVE if you need a referral to a surgeon in your area.

Treatments for Problems with Seminal Fluid

When volume of fluid is too low, medical or surgical intervention cannot correct the problem. If you have a good count, you are a candidate for artificial insemination of your own sperm (called AIH). Your sperm are separated from your own seminal fluid and resuspended in a fluid medium of the proper volume. This is then used to inseminate your partner. (A full discussion of AIH and IAIH appears in the next section.)

If you produce too much seminal fluid, a split ejaculate can be used for artificial insemination of your partner. You may elect to try withdrawal techniques for a while first before seeking further intervention, but be sure your seminal analysis shows that your first emission contains the most sperm. In some cases, the second "squirt" has more sperm.

In cases where the seminal fluid is too thick to promote good swimming conditions for the sperm, the cause could be infection. Antibiotics will be prescribed. Sometimes, doctors have tried vitamin C. But if you don't get satisfactory results, your sperm can be separated from the seminal fluid and resuspended in a more viscous fluid medium for AIH.

Antibodies present in the seminal fluid can attack and immobilize sperm. This is different from a partner immunity problem, where a woman produces antibodies to sperm. Here, a man is producing antibodies against his own sperm. This can be an immune reaction, true, but it can also result from infection or previous surgery. Have epididymitis and prostatitis (infections in the epididymis and prostate, respectively) been ruled out? When infection is found, you will be treated with antibiotics. Where an immune problem is found, your doctor may want to try lowering your immune reaction with a program of steroid therapy. This will reduce your overall immune response, so you might be left open to other infections while battling your sperm antibodies. Ask your doctor about the side effects and odds of success for this method. You may elect instead to have your sperm washed free of seminal fluid and antibodies, resuspended, and used for AIH.

Treatment for Both Partners

Artificial Insemination, Homologous (AIH, IAIH)

What Is It? AIH stands for "artificial insemination, homologous." This means artificial insemination of the woman is performed using the sperm of her own partner. In common usage, the "H" is often changed to "husband," since that's who the homologous donor usually is.

AIH may be recommended to you in hopes of overcoming a variety of problems. If the volume of semen is too low or too high, processing a man's specimen can correct the proportion of sperm to fluid. AIH, and especially its cousin IAIH (intrauterine AIH), bypasses problems of inadequate cervical mucus or sperm and mucus interaction. Sperm with poor motility or antibody problems benefit from processing and insemination. Men with low sperm counts may have a better chance on impregnating their partners if the sperm are assisted into the cervical canal or uterus, and AIH or IAIH is often suggested for them. Even in cases of impotence or retrograde ejaculation, AIH can be accomplished.

For some cases of AIH and for all case of IAIH, the man's semen is processed, or "washed," by a laboratory before it is placed in the woman's cervix or uterus. The method of processing depends on the problem at hand. Usually semen is centrifuged (spun) to separate sperm from seminal fluid. The centrifuging separates out dead sperm, malformed sperm, debris in the ejaculate, and white blood cells. The sperm can be "scrubbed" to remove antibodies. Sperm can then be resuspended in donor seminal plasma (NOT donor sperm) or in a special fluid that can help sperm fertilize the egg. Lab workers conduct sperm counts during processing to make sure the number stays as high as possible. When the sperm are squeaky clean from this washing and processing, they can be placed inside the uterus in IAIH procedures with minimal irritation and much less chance of infection. If you are concerned, you can ask the doctor or lab how the donor seminal plasma which has been donated has been screened and "sterilized" to prevent transmission of any infections or diseases.

If you are told that you are a candidate for AIH or IAIH, ask questions about why it is appropriate for you, and how it might improve your odds of conception. Processing the sperm is expensive, and you have to locate a good lab to do it. If the woman's ovulation process will be enhanced by fertility drugs (usually Clomid), what is the plan, and the cost? See what your doctor says about the number of attempts you should expect to make. How much time do you feel you have? Consider also what options may be appropriate for you in case AIH doesn't produce a pregnancy.

Things to Think About   As simple as AIH procedures appear, there are stresses associated with it for the couple starting this option. You do have to deal with a third party (your lab and doctor) intruding on what was once a natural conception process. A man who feels guilty, stigmatized, or inadequate due to his infertility may be upset that he needs another person to help him inseminate his partner. A woman may be saddened by the loss of intimacy. Together you should discuss these possibilities as you make your decisions, and you'll find that your fears will assume proper perspective. These feelings, while important, seldom block a good attitude about AIH.

A fine way to keep equilibrium is for the man to be present as his partner is inseminated. Even better, if you plan to have simple AIH with no processing, you can be quickly trained to perform the procedure at home, thus retaining your privacy. Ask about it.

The Process The woman's cycle must be carefully monitored to catch the correct day or days for insemination. This has become simpler with the urine-testing kits, but you should also be taking your BBTs. If your cycle isn't completely reliable, it may be regulated with Clomid. If fertility is to be enhanced, you may be given Clomid in combination with another fertility drug. (Take into consideration how these medications may complicate your life.)

When the day of insemination is determined, the procedure must take place within two hours after the semen specimen is produced by the man. If the semen is to be processed, you may have to rush it to the lab, or you may have to "donate" it there. The processed sperm then have to be rushed to the doctor's for immediate insemination. You can see that good planning becomes essential to orchestrate all these separate actions.

If you are bringing the specimen from home, keeping it at the proper temperature is very important. Ask your doctor to recommend the best method of transporting semen, and take into consideration how much time you need to get to the office. The "baggie in the bra" technique is favored by many: the semen is deposited into a small plastic bag that can be sealed, then tucked next to your skin—right by your heart. This keeps the semen at outside skin temperature.

At the doctor's the specimen is checked for count and volume, and then you are ready to go. For AIH, the woman lies on the regular examination table and assumes the position of a pelvic exam. After a speculum is placed in the vagina, the semen is deposited onto and slightly inside the cervical opening with a special syringe that has a curved tube. The procedure is painless. In some cases a plastic cap is placed on the cervix to keep the seminal fluid in. You'll be asked to remain lying down for fifteen to thirty minutes, giving the sperm extra time to travel. Then you can get up and resume normal activity. In six to eight hours, you can remove the cap, wash it, and save it for reuse.

IAIH is a bit more complicated. The sperm are to be deposited directly inside the uterus, shortening their travel distance and bypassing mucus. The semen specimen must be washed, so you have to factor in a fast trip to the lab first. When you arrive back at the doctor's with the processed specimen, the woman lies on the exam table as with AIH. The sperm are placed just inside the uterus with a special catheter-like device. This can cause some cramping. You may also experience some discomfort in the abdominal area. Ask your doctor what you should expect. You don't have to remain on the table, since the sperm are already in the uterus. Moving around may help the discomfort, too. Through the rest of the day, watch for any undue pain. Complications are rare, but if you do feel strange or are in pain, call your doctor.

After the first insemination, watch for the rise in your temperature that indicates ovulation has passed. In forty-eight hours, if you haven't ovulated, insemination will probably be repeated. In some cycles, women have three of them.

In the hands of caring and gentle health professionals, having AIH/IAIH is no more difficult than having a Pap smear. It's usually the tension of producing a semen specimen on demand and getting it processed in good time that can be a headache. Despite logistical problems, the prospect of success with minimal technological intervention makes AIH/IAIH a good choice for many couples.

• • •

About a week before the AIH I became very anxious and nervous. Would my husband be able to produce a sperm sample? Would I get to the office on time, or would all those little spermies die? Would the doctor get to the office on time? Would my uterus cramp up and spit out the sperm? And ... would I get pregnant?
MARGARET JOHNSON

In Vitro Fertilization (IVF)

Everyone who has read a newspaper in the last five years has heard about in vitro. The media often crudely refer to this technique as making "test tube babies," but of course this simplistic description tells us very little. IVF is the process in which surgical and medical intervention attempt to enhance and orchestrate a woman's ovulation, fertilize her egg(s) outside her body (in vitro means "in glass"), then return the fertilized embryos to her uterus to develop naturally.

IVF is being practiced by a growing number of specialists, usually in a clinic atmosphere. The fact that it has become so widespread doesn't mean it's a surefire way to become pregnant—far from it. Even the best clinics can promise only a 10 to 20 percent chance of getting a "take-home baby" from each IVF attempt. Many in vitro practices with little or no experience cannot even approach this low figure. In this light, it is necessary to learn carefully about IVF, check out prospective clinics with great care, and go in with your eyes open.

IVF may be recommended to couples as they exhaust the less invasive techniques used to enhance fertility. Couples who want every fighting chance to retain complete biological attachment to their children often consider IVF, or its cousin GIFT, before trying such alternatives as donor insemination or going on to adoption. The most common reason for trying IVF is tubal absence or damage in the woman. Fertilization occurs in the fallopian tubes, and IVF was designed to bypass them. Now even more fertility problems are considered indications for in vitro fertilization: low sperm counts, poor sperm motility, and unexplained infertility are prominent ones. Sometimes impatience on the part of the patient or the doctor may seem like a good enough reason to go for IVF, but beware.

Practical Considerations If your case makes you a candidate for IVF and you're seriously thinking about it, you face a myriad of questions about odds of success, deciphering clinic statistics, working out expenses, and logistics.

Your doctor will steer you in the direction of clinics, but you should make independent inquiries on your own. RESOLVE will send you a listing of IVF clinics. You should try to talk to one or two people who have had IVF and hear about it firsthand. As you narrow your clinic choice, this is important information to have so that you won't be surprised.

The patient selection process of most clinics has turned the prospective patient's investigative process on its head. Patients need to apply and see if they themselves are suitable. Waiting lists are a fact. These constraints may conspire to make you less picky if you find a clinic that will take you quickly, but you must try to check it out thoroughly. If you can, you must get certain basic information from the clinics. If you cannot find out anything, or the information seems vague, be careful and go elsewhere. Some of the questions you need to ask are:

- How many IVF attempts are begun by your clinic each month? (How busy is this clinic?)
- How many of these attempts result in egg retrievals? (How experienced are they in using fertility drugs?)
- How many of these initial attempts result in pregnancies each month? (Let them give you their figures for "chemical," or very early, pregnancy rate, but you need more detailed information.)
- How many of these original attempts per month result in a full-term baby? (This is the vital statistic.)
- In your clinic what is the average number of attempts needed for take-home baby success? (overall average)
- For patients with our indications, what is the average number of attempts needed for take-home baby success? (statistic best for you)
- If this attempt fails, when can we try again?
- At what point do you begin to discourage trying again?

YOUR INFERTILITY TREATMENT

- What is the training, experience, and certification of clinic doctors? How can I learn more about the doctors and staff?
- Can I contact one of your former patients?
- How long is your wait?
- What emotional support services do you provide?
- What is the scope of the auxiliary testing required beforehand?
- If I have healthy tubes, do you propose to close them? (Some do this to help their own statistics.)

What guidelines do you have as to patients' ages, general health, or infertility problems?

These dizzying questions boil down to "how much experience and training do you have, what's the take-home baby rate per month, and how long will it take us?"

As you speak with clinic representatives, don't let them snow you with statistics. Just ask firmly what these numbers translate into—can you anticipate success? Once you have established the clinic's effectiveness, you must turn your thoughts to finances. In vitro fertilization is expensive. Multiple attempts make it even more expensive. Most people have to make major budgetary adjustments to be able to afford IVF. Some people obtain loans, some even put a second mortgage on their houses. This is complicated by the refusal of some insurance companies or health-maintenance organization (HMO) plans to cover the costs of IVF. The payments made to clinics often must be made in cash (or certified check) in advance. If the cycle attempt is canceled you get only part of your money back. Pretesting and monitoring also drive up costs. You must factor in lost time from your job, and travel and accommodations if the clinic is far from home.

Insurance carriers do not like to pay for medical procedures that they consider to be experimental. Although IVF is far from a novelty anymore, the success rates are low enough for insurance companies to claim the procedure is still experimental. Check out your coverage as carefully as you can, and see if claims for the separate procedures that comprise IVF can be covered one at a time. For example, a laparoscopy can be covered as a diagnostic procedure, but perhaps not as egg retrieval for IVF. If you can, find out how other insurance companies cover IVF, and perhaps you can judiciously switch companies long before your name comes to the top of the clinic waiting list.

Only you can say if this financial hardship is worth it. If IVF succeeds, it's easy to say that of course it is, but what if it takes many attempts, and fails? It's a sobering thought, which may dampen your enthusiasm, but these are possibilities prospective IVF patients must bear in mind.

Bear in mind also the physical rigors of IVF. You'll be taking fertility drugs, probably by injection at home, having loads of blood tests, enduring ultrasounds, undergoing anesthesia, producing sperm specimens under the gun, receiving more hormones, having more blood work. Can you withstand this grueling routine, possibly from a hotel room rather than from home? Most couples find that their hope and enthusiasm carries them through these experiences, but you must thoughtfully measure how much you can take before you go ahead.

Emotional Considerations Enduring the sometimes trying circumstances of IVF attempts can be easier if you have worked hard to realistically face what's happening to you. You aren't yet ready to grieve for your biological child, but if it's still hard to accept that other couples have it so "easy," you may be depressed, angry, or resentful at the state of affairs you've found yourself in. The brusqueness of a nurse or the glibness of a doctor may really get to you. The feeling of being a cog in a big baby mill might disturb you. You'll have a less upsetting experience if you try to be as down to earth about your circumstances as possible. If you can accept that, yes, this is what it takes for us to have a baby, you'll feel stronger and determined.

But being emotionally prepared for IVF can only go so far. The suspense can be unbelievable. Will eggs mature for us? How many will we get? Will they be successfully harvested? Will they fertilize? Will they implant? Will we get pregnant? Will I be able to retain the pregnancy? Carry it to term? These questions are answered very slowly over the course of the attempt, and waiting for answers can feel like water torture.

The joy of anticipating the best results is often tempered with the thought that your attempt can end abruptly. Eggs may not mature, implantation may fail, a detected early pregnancy can be lost. Even if the clinic staff is supportive, often you will be on your own, feeling confused, frustrated, worried. Can you handle it?

With love and support from one another, couples can and do withstand this pressure, and many do quite well. But if you think you might like some additional support, locate it in advance. See what psychological professionals work with the IVF team. Call RESOLVE for a contact person you might be able to call for chats, consolation, or reassurance. Locate a support group. Often women on the same cycle timetable bond together and support each other at the clinics, but if this does not happen, knowing you can find other help is invaluable.

Ethical Considerations The process of efficient IVF attempts involves inducing several egg follicles to grow during the same month, harvesting as many as possible, and trying to fertilize them all. Placing several embryos (sometimes up to five or six) back into the uterus following fertilization and division is considered important to improve the chances of at least one or two embryos to "take," or implant, successfully. If they do implant, you are pregnant.

These practices are controversial or simply sound medical judgment, depending on your viewpoint. The question is, do those multiple embryos created in the lab dish constitute human beings? What becomes of the extra embryos? Are these embryos created only to be lost again, thus improving pregnancy odds for other embryos? Can you decide what is to be done with surplus embryos that belong to you? Can you have them frozen for the future? Do doctors conduct research on unused embryos? Is that all right? Can you donate an embryo to another childless couple? Should you try? What will happen if multiple pregnancy results?

These questions are mind-boggling. Science and technology have indeed reached beyond what our social systems can handle, so each of us must think and decide how we feel about these issues. Satisfy your own hearts and minds about these questions by reading, talking with other patients, discussing IVF with your clergyman or woman, speaking to an infertility counselor. You will probably find that your questions can be answered in a way that you can accept, and you can enter IVF feeling ready physically, emotionally, and philosophically.

The Process The search for a reputable, experienced, successful, and humane IVF clinic ends when your application for treatment is accepted. You fill out the application and forward all your relevant medical records to the clinic. Usually there is a hefty application fee. You may have to have diagnostic tests to satisfy the clinic's requirements.

There is a waiting list at most of the clinics. You can take this as a good sign—they must be doing something right, or as a bad one—how much time will we lose? Ask about the waiting period. Point out any extenuating circumstances in your case that may leapfrog you to the front of the list, such as age considerations or medical anomalies.

When your cycle attempt finally arrives, you must be in close contact with the IVF clinic because you will need attention nearly every day. For many, this means travel away from home and a hotel stay. This can be a lonely proposition, so bring some homey touches, lots of reading or work, and prepare to occupy yourselves.

Medically, you begin shortly after your new cycle has begun. Every day you will be taking fertility drugs such as Clomid tablets or Pergonal injections. You or your spouse can be quickly trained to mix the medication and give the injections. You will be monitored daily with blood work and soon, ultrasounds, to see if egg follicles are developing. Your medication may be adjusted to a different level as the days pass. You'll begin to feel the soreness from daily injections, and the suspense will begin to rise. As the time of ovulation nears, you must begin to abstain from intercourse as your doctor instructs. You will have an HCG injection to induce ovulation, and egg harvesting will proceed.

Eggs will be taken just before maturity if possible. You will have a laparoscopy under general anesthesia to remove them, or if under local anesthetic, the eggs will be aspirated with a special needle-like instrument. Ask which to expect. Avoiding general anesthetic is usually a good idea, but the doctor will advise you.

The eggs are taken and examined for their condition. The good eggs are placed in a dish with a fluid that promotes their maturity. In the meantime, the man is asked to produce a semen specimen, which will be processed for optimum chances of fertilization. The sperm and eggs are mixed in the lab dish at the proper time and are allowed some hours for fertilization. If fertilization is seen, more time is given for the cells to develop and begin division, usually a day or two.

In the next procedure, the fertilized eggs (now embryos) are placed in a catheter, and are then deposited into the uterus. This could cause some cramping, but it is essentially a simple procedure. You'll rest for a few hours at the clinic, then you will be able to leave. Bed rest is usually ordered for the remainder of the day and for the following day.

More tests of your blood hormone levels come next, and you may be given progesterone to assist implantation and support of the early pregnancy. Then you wait until it's time for your pregnancy test.

This time of the cycle can be a killer. You've come so far already. Your hopes are soaring, yet sometimes you think you dare not hope. The days can pass so slowly. But finally a blood test will reveal if you have a "chemical" or very early pregnancy. At this stage you may be pregnant, but unfortunately, you are still in some danger of losing it. About 15 percent of IVF embryos fail to implant at all. About 25 percent to 30 percent of the early pregnancies spontaneously abort before the first missed period, and some 10 percent may miscarry later in the pregnancy. The odds are improving, but until science understands the natural mechanisms of pregnancy more fully and learns to imitate them better, many IVF attempts will, sadly, be hit-and-miss.

Pregnancies that succeed via IVF are closely watched. You'll probably have an amniocentesis. Keep in mind that lots of IVF babies are delivered by Caesarean section, so check this out ahead of time. Having a C-section should be a negotiable point if you're having a normal pregnancy.

If your IVF attempt fails this time, you will feel sad and tired, and perhaps angry. The clinic will let you know when you can try again, but usually after this you are on your own to cope with the disappointment. Think carefully about what your goals are, your energy resources, your finances, and especially your emotional reserves, and listen to your heart. Deciding to go again is courageous and life-affirming, and most doctors agree that couples usually need more than one try. But there is no shame in deciding to turn to another alternative if you find that IVF is not right for you. No matter which way you go, you can find love and support to see you through.

Gamete Intra-Fallopian Transfer (GIFT)

GIFT is a variation of in vitro fertilization that has developed and that is finding a receptive clientele. It is cheaper and somewhat more natural than IVF, but the woman must have at least one intact fallopian tube. As in IVF, the woman is given fertility drugs, and has her eggs harvested when they mature. The eggs are harvested during a laparoscopy, conducted under general anesthesia. Instead of transferring the eggs to a dish to be fertilized, the doctors mix the man's processed sperm specimen with the eggs right at this moment, and then place the mixture into the fallopian tubes. If the eggs are going to be fertilized, they do it on their own, out of sight of medical science. The embryos travel to the uterus and implant by themselves. It is hoped that this more natural approach encourages these processes.

GIFT is considered a breakthrough for women who have intact tubes but have endometriosis, mucus problems, a partner with a poor sperm count, or unexplained infertility. It is less expensive than IVF because two procedures (egg monitoring and fertilization, and embryo transfer) are eliminated, and because laparoscopies can usually be insured. It eliminates some of that man-made suspense, since you will not know if the eggs are fertilized or have implanted until a pregnancy test can be done.

Before the actual egg harvesting and GIFT procedure, the egg follicles are stimulated with fertility drugs as described for IVF. The woman is given the drug to develop multiple follicles, she gets an HCG shot before ovulation, and the GIFT process ensues.

Finding a clinic to perform GIFT should follow the same guidelines as finding IVF centers. Most clinics doing IVF do GIFT, but practices vary. Finding the right clinic is so important because the administration of fertility drugs and anesthesia, and the orchestration of reproduction require skill, experience, and humanity. This cannot be emphasized enough.

If you've been told you are a candidate for IVF but you think you qualify for GIFT, do ask about it. Ask about success rates, take-home baby rates, and how the clinic procedure will go, just as you would for IVF. Be well aware that results and statistics are sketchy, and that this procedure is even younger than IVF, whose success rates are still low after many years. Use RESOLVE's contact system and talk to a GIFT veteran—they are a growing number.

With a Full Bladder and Your Heart in Your Throat

JENNIFER MILFORD

I think that everyone has had a nightmare similar to the one in which you find yourself in a class, taking an exam that you didn't study for. That's as close as I can describe the feeling of preparing for my GIFT surgery.

After passing a preliminary exam at the start of a cycle, you go home and give yourself injections and pills until the eighth day, when the real tests start. Then you present yourself each morning for testing to see if your body is doing the right thing. Passing or failing means everything. You sit in the waiting room with a full bladder for ultrasound and your heart in your throat. The faces of the other women begin to look familiar and you begin to talk. Each of you waits for the fantastic announcement that surgery will be tomorrow, and you hope you aren't told to come back next cycle. Every day, every injection brings you one step closer to the final exam that you have prayed so hard to pass.

Slowly the number of women you know dwindles as they drop out or have surgery. Finally your turn comes and you go back in the late evening for a final test and injection, and even then everything could be canceled. When it isn't, you face something even more frightening, the true possibility that you have reached the end, the ultimate attempt at pregnancy.

So many years have gone by, full of cycles that held promise, yet for each one you reserved a small space of self-survival, called doubt. It was too hard to keep believing and it hurt too much when the bleeding started, so you kept the small secret sentence inside and repeated, "I don't think I'm pregnant." Now the big push is on, and you have to believe because you've staked all your hopes and dreams on this, and there's no place else to go. You can't even allow the thought of another time, another month, because this is it.

All I did was all that I could do, which was believe that I would finally hear the words I had rehearsed in my mind for so long: "You're pregnant."

Pregnancy After Infertility

Becoming pregnant after a bout with infertility is what all of us dream of. Many men and women have daydreams (and night dreams, too) in which the happy moment is enacted in its most perfect scenario: "Congratulations! You're going to be parents!"

For some people, this dream is the fuel that keeps them going. It's difficult to tackle tests, medication, timed sex, or surgery without a dream like this to spur you on. It's also a source of escape and comfort.

When you become pregnant, the dream meets reality. Some couples are able to grasp the news and feel great happiness and relief. Some will react with some degree of disbelief. You have spent months or years struggling along, and suddenly the struggle is over. It can come as a shock, no matter how earnestly this pregnancy was longed for. You may find yourself asking, "Is this really happening?" All couples have to switch gears from the "we're infertile" mentality to the "we're expecting!" mentality.

How you react and cope with your pregnancy can to some extent depend on how you coped with your infertility. If you were a worrier before, you may feel anxious now about your pregnancy. It has come at a high emotional price, and you may not be able to turn off your "worry" faucet right away. You might be concerned that you could miscarry. This might be a justifiable worry, or it could be that you're just used to expressing anxiety connected with your ability to reproduce. If you are worried for either reason, it's time to get your questions in hand and deal with them so you can enjoy your pregnancy. Talk to your infertility specialist again, and to your obstetrician. Have them talk to each other, too. Find out if you have any basis for concern. You can go over the section in this book on miscarriage, and use it as a jumping-off point in your discussions. Any health-related question you may have about yourself or your baby should never be left unasked.

If you "bargained" in your mind to become more deserving of your pregnancy, you may now feel somehow that it's time to "pay up." You might as a result not feel entitled to complain about morning sickness, high obstetrical fees, or other of the normal concerns expectant parents have. You may keep to yourself your worry about the baby's health, you may feel badly that you'll miss your two-someness as a couple when your baby is born. Sometimes your family or friends may actually shush you if you voice these perfectly normal feelings, thinking that after all you've been through, how can you complain now?

What you need to remember is that all expectant parents have these feelings, and that's why you have them, too! All parents-to-be worry, are elated, wonder about their parenting abilities at times, get scared. You are just as entitled as they are to these emotions. Your struggle to have this baby doesn't take away your very human, natural reactions to this event.

As you've come through your experience of infertility, you may have discovered other friends with the same problem. Or you may have become friendly with infertile couples at RESOLVE meetings, at the doctor's, in a support group, at the IVF clinic. When you succeed at becoming pregnant, you might find yourself feeling a little bit guilty around these friends. Sometimes your friends will have mixed emotions towards you, and this is something you have to understand and accept. Yes, they are happy for you, but yes, they are also envious. Some men and women feel that they have in some sense "graduated " and left their friends behind. You may not have felt this way since adolescence, when you and your friends began menstruating, wearing makeup, shaving, or dating at different times. Sharing your pregnancy with these infertile friends can be a bittersweet experience. You will probably feel sad if you find you are growing apart as your interests diverge. If your friendship is genuine, it will survive this somewhat rough time. But if all you and your friend had in common was your infertility, it may be hard to maintain your relationship. Empathy and warm regard for one another will always help.

As you progress through your pregnancy and project into your future as parents, don't give yourself the added burden of perfection. After infertility, it can be easy to think that everything has to be done just right with your baby, because this may be your only chance. Or, after having your pregnancy deferred, you may want to dote on this baby and indulge it. Natural feelings, to be sure! But you and your child need a chance to be regular, ordinary people, too. Being overprotective and spoiling your child is such a natural tendency, but try to keep it in perspective. One of your great challenges as your child grows will be your ability to gradually let it go out into the world and take chances. Every kid needs to do it, and a child born of formerly-infertile parents is no different.

Having given all this cautionary advice, there is one thing left to say: it's time for you both to clamber up to the nearest rooftop and scream and shout your heads off! Congratulations! You're going to be parents!

Does This Mean My Infertility Is Resolved?

MARGIE GERETY

*A*lthough I am seven months pregnant, I still consider myself an infertile person. Once a person has gone through so much pain and agony, so many ups and downs, it is difficult to consider yourself fertile. Does getting pregnant this time mean my infertility is resolved? Will God bless me with another miracle if we should want another child? Will this child be born healthy, or did we use up all of our good luck getting pregnant? The pain of infertility does not immediately disappear with a positive pregnancy test. I still keep waiting to wake up and find that it was all a dream.

I have quite a few friends who have been trying to have a baby for years. Many have tried so much longer than I did, and I can feel their envy when I am near them. The resentment is there, although it is not obvious—I know because I went through it, too. I felt those feelings of hate that you can't seem to help having. One of my closest friends had a hysterectomy seven years ago. I know she is unhappy to be childless, but she has faced the fact and has focused on other interests. I can see that it is much easier for her to deal with and be genuinely happy for me. It is hard not to center my whole life and my conversations around this baby, but I let my infertile friends bring up the subject first.

Even after you think your infertility is resolved, there is still much to think about. My husband and I are working hard to stop being paranoid at every ache and pain. It will be a challenge not to be overprotective parents. Once you are infertile it's hard to break away from those fears. Although very pregnant, I can still feel for others who are infertile—even more now that I know what they are missing.

I Was Looking at a Stranger

JUDY BRADSHAW

I was like any other infertile woman, daydreaming what it would be like to find out I was pregnant. My husband and I would have indescribable joy, and live happily ever after. So many friends and family prayed for a pregnancy to happen, and two months before my thirty-sixth birthday, it did. I experienced many emotions, but joy wasn't one of them. I had a positive pregnancy test when I went in for my pre-op exam for a scheduled myomectomy to remove a fibroid. This time the positive was for real, after suffering a false positive two months before.

My specialist was delighted, as were family and friends. Everybody except me. I was convinced my body was playing another cruel joke on me. Six days later I started cramping and spotting. I cried because I was sure it was all over. An ultrasound and HCG test proved otherwise, but the ultrasound showed the baby precariously close to the fibroid. That, and my luteal phase defect, could have caused a miscarriage.

The spotting continued for some time, and I was afraid to plan for the baby. I read of a woman who had been infertile and was so numb that she couldn't plan for her baby. Her mother and sister had to do the nursery for her. When her water broke, her husband told her it was time to go to the hospital. She asked, "Why?" I could relate to this. I couldn't take any presents out of their packages until after my son was born. I couldn't go into maternity shops because I was late in showing and the clerks would ask me whom I was shopping for. I ascribed my pregnancy symptoms to other causes. I was nauseated and gaining weight because of too much junk food. I was always tired because I was lazy.

Another unexpected emotion I had to deal with was guilt. I have made friends with many other infertiles. How could I tell them? Why me and not them? They deserved a baby more. I couldn't look at other pregnant women. When I looked at my own pregnant form in the mirror, I was looking at a stranger. Every new pregnancy, baby, or shower at church still brought the same old pain. I hardly remember my own shower. Nobody wanted to hear about the problems I was having. They all reminded me of all the times I thought I would never get pregnant. Fertile women get sympathy, I thought, and I get criticism.

The spotting stopped, but the nightmares began. I was still bleeding in these dreams, or the baby had something wrong with it. Or I had the baby, but nobody at the hospital could tell me where it was.

My fertility specialist and my obstetrician are in the same building, and my husband had to steer me away from the specialist's office toward the obstetrician's. I had invested so much time and energy there, I really missed the specialist and his staff. I still do.

I finally started to relax and enjoy the pregnancy during the seventh month, because I realized that the baby could survive if born then. All too soon the last two months were over. I hated to put away the maternity clothes—I had been cheated out of the first seven months.

My son is two months old now, and the joy that eluded me for most of the pregnancy is building every day. Old hurts still surface, but they are easier to handle now.

SECTION IV
The Alternatives

*M*any couples going through the experience of infertility are curious about the different ways it can be resolved. Medical treatments can bring pregnancy with one partner retaining biological attachments, or children can be adopted. Certain special couples can decide to become childfree.

You may need help in finding out what alternatives could suit you best. You may need help in just thinking and talking about them. This section will give you a head start.

You will find descriptions of the alternatives that allow couples to retain partial biological attachment to their children. You can read about the practical, emotional, and ethical considerations that you need to think about when you try these alternatives on for size. Plus, you can learn about what to do if you think adoption suits your needs. Also included here are some facts of life about what each alternative can—and cannot—do for you.

Reading through this section should give you a realistic sense of hope. There are so many things that you can do to resolve infertility. This is indeed an experience that you can come to terms with, and it's one you can use to strengthen yourselves and your relationship. As you bring this chapter of your life to a close, you'll have bittersweet memories, of course. But if you work now to find the right choices for yourselves, you can begin to see this experience in a new perspective—as a very meaningful, and ultimately rewarding, time of your life.

Look Ahead to Choices

Life events ought to take place in some logical, understandable order. But that isn't the case very often. This fact of life can be emphasized as you live through the events of infertility—getting help, being tested, being treated, building your family. These phases can seem to happen in a jumble, out of sequence, hardly giving you a chance to think clearly about what you're doing.

Part of the reason things may seem out of kilter is that even as you get help and make decisions, you're caught in emotional turmoil. There are times you feel energetic and determined, and other times when you feel despair. In this book, finding help with some sense of logic is the main goal, but preparing for future actions and choices is important, too.

Options are what this section is all about. Happily, there are plenty of alternatives to consider as you look ahead. Some options are controversial, some are expensive, some are traditional. All deserve careful thought and a lot of looking before leaping.

The circumstances surrounding each infertile couple are different. You may wonder, "Why do we have to decide anything now? We aren't ready." Remember, you don't have to make any decision you don't feel ready for. Even if you feel you are up against the clock, you need time to think and to progress emotionally toward the solution that's right for you.

Some couples do wish to look ahead because the existence of alternatives can be reassuring to them. Beyond the natural, dual-biological parenting that we initially consider most desirable, there are other ways to build a family. We can also examine our innermost goals as best we can, and consider living a full, childfree life. And we learn that whatever way we go, we can finally begin to feel a sense of resolution—at last.

Talking About Your Alternatives

When you start wondering which family-building option may be right for you, remember two things. First, informing yourself about your choices is the best way to be sure you're making a good decision. Secondly, frank communication with your partner is absolutely essential.

To start off, your own medical case will guide you toward your special needs. Your doctor probably has already suggested which alternatives could work for you. When you understand your case by participating closely in your workups and treatments, you'll readily see which way your path may take you.

Arm yourself with as much information as you can. Read medical books, talk to friends, read popular magazines, call RESOLVE, interview medical personnel, or talk to adoption workers. The more you can learn, the more confidence you'll have in your ultimate decision. The alternative that initially appeals to you could pale as you get the inside story from a veteran. By the same token, a method you never seriously considered could grow in your estimation because erroneous beliefs about it are dispelled by accurate information. Knowing too much isn't going to scare you away from a decision if it's the right decision for you.

Don't take for granted your communication skills as a couple. You can discuss any and all possibilities together in an open, nonthreatening atmosphere. Talking about an alternative doesn't mean you have to commit yourself to it. Knock around your wildest fears, deepest hopes, most important needs. You each need to take responsibility for accurately stating your own point of view, and clarifying it for your partner. You must give a full hearing to your partner's viewpoint and ask for clarification yourself. Don't assume you know. Don't assume your partner knows. It's a trap couples can fall into.

Be forthright. Be as frank as you can. State how you feel yourself, and let your ideas stand for themselves. Don't state your feelings as a comparison to your partner's. Don't be threatened if your partner doesn't agree with you—you are only in the preliminary stages of making a decision, so don't feel defensive.

If you're just not sure how you feel, state that, too. Your ambivalent feelings are also legitimate indicators of what's happening with you, and your partner needs to know them. Your partner has ambivalences, too—we all do.

After preliminary "think tank" talks together about alternatives, spend some more time gathering information. Learn what you can, and be sure to share your information with your partner. Don't do it to coerce or even persuade. Information is strength all by itself, no matter what decisions come from it. Later you can come back to a more specific discussion of your views, based on what you now know. Can you see an agreement coming along? Is there compromise possible?

Good compromises for couples who have not made an ironclad decision are the "in the meantime" ones. If one of you is moving toward adoption, you can place your name on agency waiting lists in the meantime. If IVF may be in your future, you can try AIH, and in the meantime get on an in vitro program's waiting list. Layering your options keeps you confident that even while you decide, you are not standing still and losing time.

But do give yourselves time to get into synchronization. Your relationship consists of two separate heads and hearts. Even if your time is running out on certain options, try to give yourselves some slack. Periodically remind yourselves, in a nonthreatening, objective way, of your deadline, then reopen discussions and restate your views.

If you hit a wall and cannot agree, if your relationship is showing the strain of your differences, if you're beginning to panic because you fear you'll never work it out, consider a few sessions with a counselor. Having a third party objectively mediate will throw your talks into a new dimension, and may speed compromise along. A counselor specializing in infertility is trained to help couples over these rough patches. If you're putting off deciding because you're afraid you'll choose the wrong option and regret it later, a counselor will help you deal with this anxiety. Any important decision carries this worry within it. There are regrets connected to any road not taken, but if you carefully decide with full information, you have little to fear.

Once you hit upon a compromise or fully agree, your energy and enthusiasm will increase as you move toward implementing your decision. In a short while, you may wonder what in the world you were so worried about. Your confidence will rise, and you'll feel ready for the challenge ahead. Good luck.

The Need to Grieve

Grief is a normal, natural human process of reacting to and gradually accepting the loss of a loved one. It is well understood that the bereaved need to experience grief in order to be better able to grasp their loss and become able to go on with their lives. Infertility, however, is sometimes a state of limbo in terms of grief. Couples experiencing infertility are often reluctant to acknowledge that there's any reason to grieve at all. Family and friends may also skirt around infertility and not see it as a loss. In fact, as you read this you may be wondering why and how the issue of grief even applies to your situation.

If you find out you can't have your biological child, this is a loss. Sometimes couples are told suddenly that there is little hope. More likely, couples keep trying, with just one more month's worth of energy and optimism keeping them going. Some doctors may also be reluctant to throw in the towel and can encourage couples to keep trying. Some couples try beyond a reasonable chance of success, but can't recognize it.

How do you know if it is time to move on? You may begin to feel very tired of medical treatment or begin to lose sight of your goals. One day you may notice that you're having many more bad days than good days. It can slowly (or quickly) dawn on you that it's time to get busy thinking about alternatives. These feelings may be telling you that you're ready to consider new ideas, plans, decisions.

It may be hard to let go of your old patterns of coping and living with infertility. Coming out on the other side of grief helps change your thinking. Grief will free you to think about your options without the feeling of panic or the overwhelming sense of loss that can cloud your judgment. It will help you to determine your goals and desires about children, your life, your relationship. It can clarify your values.

Grieving for your lost biological child sounds like an abstract concept. There is no tangible loss, except in your hearts and dreams. Nobody else sees or experiences this feeling as you do, and often, as a result, you might not get the support you need. Plus, if you are finally forced (by emotional or physical reasons) to end medical treatment, you might feel guilty about "pulling the plug." For all these reasons, you may resist grief.

Embracing grief is a scary prospect, but it doesn't mean that you are giving up or that you are a failure. It means that you are learning to accept certain facts about your life.

How can a person start grieving after holding in painful feelings for so long? Opening up to full grief is frightening. After many months when you have experienced cycles of hope followed by despair, you may legitimately feel you're already grieving. The sadness and disappointment you felt when a menstrual period arrived or a treatment didn't succeed was a "mini" grief, but it was always tempered by your rising hopes for the next month or the next treatment. Now there is no next month or next treatment.

The pain you've felt month after month may be so intense that you fear you'll go out of control—or crazy—should you allow yourselves to fully grieve. This does not happen. If you've been coping by withdrawing or just numbing out, bringing grief to the surface might be a problem. You may not know how to grieve.

Barbara Eck Menning, RESOLVE's founder, has been an infertility counselor for many years. She has recognized that grief may fail to come forth for some infertile people, and they need to be helped to face their emotions. They need encouragement and especially support so they can allow their very strong feelings to be expressed.

In most cases, you can help each other by calling to a halt all the defenses you have used to keep mourning at bay. You must no longer use your dreams and imagination to picture what your child would have been like, how your family life would have been, and think that this specific scenario will probably never come true for you. Yes, you are now allowed to feel sorry for yourself that this has happened. You are entitled. Force yourself to dwell on poignant details that you've deliberately avoided thinking about in the past. This will help to bring your feelings to the surface.

If you are unsure that you will be able to do this "grief work," seeking the short-term help of a trained counselor may help you. If you get stuck, these professionals will be able to help you to work out your feelings.

What will grief be like? Some of us have already experienced the loss of loved ones and have learned about grief this way. But to many people with infertility problems, this may be one of the first major losses of their lives.

The pain and sense of emptiness you've felt in the past will probably return more intensely as you grieve fully. You will cry, you will feel deep despair, you will feel anger, guilt, depression, confusion, loneliness. If you allow yourselves to feel these emotions and keep telling yourself that yes, this is really happening, your grief process will progress. It will gradually play itself out and come to an end. Give it time. Unfortunately, you will probably have to keep going to work and holding your life together, but try to give yourselves as much latitude as possible.

You will come out of your grief and regain interest in living, social activities, and your work. You'll begin to exhibit interest and enthusiasm in building a new life in new ways. Alternatives will cease to threaten you but will instead present exciting possibilities. You won't forget completely what this feeling of loss is like, but it will begin to hurt you less intensely. You will have "relapses," to which you are fully entitled; it doesn't mean you are weak. But you will find you are feeling stronger and more optimistic, and you'll realize that these positive feelings are going to stay with you.

Imaginary Child

BONNIE WEBSTER

I close my eyes
I see you near me

I hold you close
We both can feel it

You touch my cheek
And remove a tear

I open my eyes
And you disappear.

Considering Alternatives: The Best Interests of . . . Whom?

As you learn about the family-building options that are best for you, don't forget to think about what you feel will be best for your baby.

You can start by reconsidering your motives for wanting a child. Knowing which alternatives are medically indicated for you can be balanced against your fundamental desires for parenting. How important is it to retain partial genetic attachment? Do you want the experience of pregnancy if at all possible? Do you just love kids and want some? Do you think children make life complete, or can you channel your nurturing needs elsewhere and choose to live childfree? Are you constrained by religious, moral, or ethical questions? Are you feeling panicked and just want a child, no matter what it takes?

How do you view parenting? In terms of blood ties, or in terms of rearing a child? Do you feel a child develops and grows according to nature or to nurturing? In twenty years, will it even matter what method you chose to build your family? Does joyous anticipation of parenthood outweigh possible misgivings when you think of the tasks ahead? Do you focus on the result (a child or children) or on the processes used to obtain it?

How is your relationship doing? The best interests of any child include what atmosphere the child is brought into. Do you think you still have unresolved or unexplored feelings about your infertility to deal with? While no one completely gets over infertility forever, you should feel that you are making a good start. If you hurry up and adopt or hurry up and have AID (artificial insemination supplied by a donor), your emotional needs may crop up later, when you're trying to cope with parenthood, too.

Do you feel children will cement your relationship? That's a heavy burden to give to a child. Is there a possibility of guilt feelings or feelings of inadequacy if one parent is not genetically connected to the baby? Are either of you accustomed to "going along" with the desires of the other? Could this be happening as you try to resolve your infertility?

Now, switch gears from considering your needs and think about your prospective child. Use your imagination and conjure up him or her as a human presence as you consider its best interests, its feelings, its needs. Will what you do now have any real effect on your child? Will you feel able to help your child handle the realities of its origin, whatever that origin turns out to be?

How do you feel about openness, honesty, secrecy? Some of the alternatives will certainly provoke these questions. What do you feel is your child's right to know? How can you explain things in a way that keeps the child feeling as loved and wanted as possible? If you elect for secrecy, will it hang over your heads your entire life, or can it be dismissed and forgotten?

If your chosen alternative involves a third party, how will you deal with her or him? Do you feel it is necessary to retain absolute anonymity or can you live with open acknowledgment of this person? Is there a compromise that you both can live with?

The media are swirling with reports on the large ethical questions surrounding certain family-building methods, but interestingly, the pain that brings couples to these alternatives is rarely mentioned, and the joy that results from their successful utilization is never mentioned. Don't be overly influenced by what you may be reading in the papers. Find other couples who have gone through what you are about to try, and hear about their experiences. A secure decision, made after hearing the facts and by considering the issues raised by these facts, will build your confidence and free you to enjoy your child.

Artificial Insemination, Donor (AID)

Artificial insemination using sperm supplied by a donor other than the spouse, AID for short, is very common. Thousands of children are born each year using this alternative method of family building. While it's pretty simple technically, there are emotional, ethical, legal, and religious questions that couples should bear in mind as they consider AID.

AID is recommended by doctors when the male partner of an infertile couple is known to have a genetic problem, has a very low sperm count (called oligospermia), or poor motility, or produces no sperm. Some men request AID because of their previous exposure to hazardous chemicals, toxics, or radiation. If medication or surgery has produced little realistic hope for conception, the couple may wish to turn to AID in order to retain partial genetic continuity with the child, or to provide the woman with the experience of pregnancy.

If talk of AID is cropping up in your discussions with your doctor, bear in mind that finding a significant infertility problem in the man does not always mean the woman is problem-free. Don't abruptly break off your workup until the major factors in female infertility are checked and eliminated.

In some cases, AIH/IAIH may be tried before turning to AID. Ask your specialist if there's a reasonable chance for this approach. Some cases are also candidates for IVF or GIFT. If complete genetic attachment to your baby is very important, explore those options carefully. They are far more expensive and taxing than AID, and the failure rate can be high. If you can accept the need for a sperm donor, AID is technologically much simpler.

Many couples find that after consideration, AID is more than acceptable as an alternative. It retains partial genetic continuity, allows the couple to experience pregnancy, birth, and breastfeeding, and gives a couple the chance to parent from birth. The trepidations couples can experience usually evaporate once they have done grief work and have accepted their situation. When the baby arrives, they wonder what the fuss was all about. The real work is the initial job of figuring out if AID is right for you.

Emotional Considerations

With AID, as with the prospect of any family-building option, it is important to come to terms with your situation. You may have to grieve for the loss of a biological child who is attached to you genetically on both sides. You must accept the loss of something you hoped to accomplish together—creating your baby. Full realization of this fact will often trigger a period of grieving, which is normal and necessary. Coming through this emotion clears your thinking and helps you deal logically with the tasks that await you as you choose this alternative.

In addition to this loss, each partner must individually come to terms with the man's infertility and the wife's fertility. The man may feel guilty or inadequate at first. He may fear being "left out" of the process as AID is attempted. He must fully accept that another man's sperm may impregnate his partner and give them their child. It can be helpful to consider AID as a chance to adopt your child early by adopting half its genetic makeup—it's like adopting the sperm.

The woman may feel guilty that she was untouched by this problem. Why was it him and not me? She must allow herself to feel sorry that she can't bear her partner's child, and not cover up this regret to soften the blow for the man. She should allow her partner to feel his loss fully and not rush him into accepting AID before he is ready.

Sometimes the woman may feel strange about being impregnated with the sperm of another man, an anonymous donor. She may need reassurance from her partner, when he is ready to give it. His presence at all insemination attempts is highly desirable, and helps both partners make the prospective conception their very own.

If you are very anxious to get started on AID right away, can you say why? Don't rush into it as a way to quickly mask your infertility and make it go away. This may mean that you haven't accepted your problem yet. And don't "go along" with AID just to please your partner or atone for some perceived transgression. Going into AID without full enthusiastic participation of both partners is not a good idea. Take some time to examine your goals, your feelings, your motives.

In fact, pre-AID counseling with a qualified professional isn't a bad idea. A conscientious specialist will urge you to try counseling. It doesn't mean you can't make your own decisions or that you're crazy. Counseling can scope out any possible problems connected with AID, and inform you about what you can expect. You will really feel ready if you have done this kind of preparation.

Practical Considerations

Secrecy and AID The burning issue that crops up after you decide to try AID is that of secrecy. And secrecy itself has many aspects: how much you want to know about your donor, how many people will know the donor's identity, if the medical records will be available and to whom, and what the child should know—all are considerations.

Your doctor will probably handle locating and screening the donor that is appropriate for you. The donor's identity will be kept from you, and yours from him. The doctor knows both, so she must have your trust in her screening methods and criteria. After they are fully explained to you, are you satisfied? Ask any question, no matter how strange it sounds. If you feel uncomfortable surrendering this much control to your doctor, you should continue to question if AID is right for you.

Even though the identity of your donor is secret, there should be assurances of lifelong access to the donor's medical history, just in case. Be sure that the records will not be destroyed. Keeping the medical details from you isn't secrecy—it's withholding vital information that you may need someday. The records can be sealed, they can bear no name, but they should be available.

Another issue of secrecy is who you feel should know that you are having AID. Your family? Your friends? Your child? If so, how do you convey this information, and when? What will you say?

There is a wide trend towards "open" adoption, where the birth parents are known to the adoptive parents, and sometimes to the adoptee as well. Children or young adult adoptees can request meetings with their birth parents. There is reason to assume that some people will extend this attitude to the donors for AID. This is uncharted territory, and if you are considering this idea, proceed with the utmost caution.

What do you believe are the child's rights to its heritage? What do you believe a child can handle? Can you pretend you are a child receiving this news? How will you talk about such matters to a four-year-old, or later, when the child is seven, ten, fifteen, twenty-one?

What do you see as the rights of the donor? Some men may feel curious if their donation "worked," while others just donate and forget it. Most would not be prepared to reveal their identity and have a child knock on the door someday. If you tell the child of its heritage but then cannot supply its father's name, this is not fair either, so tread carefully.

If you tell family or friends but don't want the child to know, will secrecy be possible over many years? Would you want this knowledge to be in the air but never mentioned? Or would you prefer to keep a lock on the information and not tell anyone? Families or friends may not react to AID the way you want them to, so deviating from a policy of total secrecy may be risky.

If you keep this fact between just yourselves, you'll have control over it. It won't hang over your heads your whole lives, as many AID parents can assure you. The fact that you used a donor will dissolve over time, and you will not feel like you're sitting on a time bomb. You have to make a leap of faith on this point, but your faith will be well served.

Screening Donors Screening prospective donors has entered a new dimension with the widespread incidence of sexually transmitted diseases, infections, acquired immune deficiency syndrome, and the use of drugs. More care than ever is being taken to see that a donor is not only genetically and medically sound, but that his lifestyle isn't exposing him to further risk. This is especially necessary if AID is performed with fresh instead of frozen semen. For your protection ask about how the fresh semen is processed.

The donation process begins with the donor filling out a long questionnaire detailing the specific health and medical history of family members. It usually runs back to three generations. The health of the donor's siblings and children, if any, is documented. An extensive genetic assay, or karyotype, is not usually done because it is very expensive. If there are special circumstances in your case, it can be requested.

More subjective criteria come into play in selecting a donor. How intelligent is the donor? What seem to be his natural talents? What is his chosen career? Does he have a pleasant personality? Sometimes prospective AID parents consider these factors just as important as matching the physical characteristics of the donor to the father. If you have questions like these, even if you think they might be considered odd, you should ask your doctor anyway. If the donor is known to the doctor personally or professionally, you might get your answers.

Using Fresh or Frozen Sperm Another practical problem is choosing to use fresh or frozen sperm for AID. Fresh sperm is of better quality and has a higher pregnancy rate, and it is less expensive. However, fresh samples mean the donor must be on call and able to produce two or three specimens per woman per cycle. If you are using a donor near a medical education center or hospital, this might work out well. Fresh semen cannot be given the extensive testing or screening for infection, count, or sperm motility before it is used for insemination. However, if the donor has been thoroughly screened, tests on recent samples should reassure you that the man is healthy and producing good sperm. Plus, if the donor is reliable enough to show up at odd times to donate, his medical history and health can probably be trusted, too. Get reassurance from the doctor for any questions you have, especially if the semen is not being processed prior to insemination.

Frozen sperm is more expensive, and it may offer reduced motility and lower counts per sample. But frozen sperm comes from sperm banks, and you are able to choose from a wider pool of donors. The frozen sperm specimens can be examined and screened for infection or disease. They can be obtained at odd times, sometimes with the help of expensive delivery services.

Your doctor probably has a preference for one form over the other. If your doctor uses fresh samples only, find out why she feels that way. You can call RESOLVE for information on sperm banking if you want to know more.

Paperwork The last practical hurdle is straightening out the legal paperwork. There are varying laws from state to state, so no rule of thumb applies to AID. Your doctor, who has experience with these matters, can help guide you. You can protect yourselves by preparing a consent form that can be signed by both of you and perhaps witnessed by the doctor. In this form, you state your knowledge and understanding of the AID process, absolve the donor and the doctor of liability, and state that the child will be supported by you as your legitimate heir.

Your doctor may be able to steer you to legal advice, but you can ask RESOLVE for referrals if you can't find a lawyer with this type of experience. With a qualified family lawyer you can hash out such issues as the fate of the donor's medical records, assuring anonymity, and so on.

The Process

The woman monitors her cycle by using a urine-testing kit and by taking her temperature. It is sometimes helpful for the man to take charge of the temperature records, so both partners feel involved with even this preliminary stage of AID.

When ovulation seems imminent, you notify the doctor, and arrangements are made to obtain the fresh or frozen sperm. In the doctor's office the woman lies on the examination table as if for a pelvic exam. After placement of a speculum in the vagina, a special syringe will bathe the cervix with semen. You will be told to remain lying down for about half an hour. In some cases a small plastic cup will cap your cervix to keep the semen in place. This can be removed in six to eight hours, washed, and kept for future inseminations.

After telling you to stay on the examination table for a while, the medical professional will probably leave, as there are other patients to see. Having your partner along for the insemination process makes particular sense at this point in the process. These can be precious moments together, at an important time in your relationship. If job responsibilities conspire to keep you apart, be prepared

THE ALTERNATIVES

with a little light reading or even a small tape player with headphones. It's no fun to count the holes in the acoustic ceiling tile right after such a momentous event.

Watch for your temperature rise, indicating ovulation has passed. Ask your doctor for guidelines, but if your temperature doesn't rise promptly, you'll go back for another insemination in thirty-six to forty-eight hours.

It usually takes three to six cycles for AID to work. You have to be patient and give your body a chance to work. In some cases, doctors advocate enhancing fertility with medication in conjunction with AID. See what your doctor says.

When you become pregnant it is natural to have certain fears about the baby's appearance, intelligence, health. All parents-to-be have these worries. Many AID parents report a big sigh of relief when they give birth to healthy, sound children, and their anxieties disappear. Plan on the fullest joint participation in the birth process as you can manage, which will help both parents feel a sense of belonging and of wonderment that is special indeed.

I Must Tell Someone

JENNIFER LUND

i sat quietly in the car as we drove to the first of many fertility tests, thinking that it would be easier to deal with if it were me instead of him. I was wrong in so many ways.

My husband is an extremely private person, whereas I usually feel better when telling it all. Unfortunately, the results of our postcoital test are not something I can tell all. My husband was found to be azoospermic.

In our society when something fails, someone is at fault. So it is with the fertile population; when faced with an infertile couple, they want to know whose "fault" it is. What they don't know is that both face a feeling of incompleteness, and to point a finger at one of us only deepens the despair. Even if my husband wouldn't mind the disclosure, I cannot admit his inability to father our children. Would he be blamed, his masculinity, his sexual prowess put in question? So I have taken full responsibility for our childlessness. My inability to conceive with AID fosters this acceptance. I explain my doctor's visits with vague references to "medication" that must be administered by my doctor and the necessity of closely monitoring my faulty ovulation.

I shrug my shoulders when questions become specific and nod vigorously when asked by slightly more knowledgeable people, "Does his sperm count check out OK?"

I wish it were different. I wish I could explain in the detail I would like. I wish I were pregnant. I wish that when I speak of my inability to conceive, I could be honest. Instead, when I explain my infertility to others, I lie.

It is so difficult to deal with the emotion I face monthly as I purchase someone's sperm and lie in an office while it is placed inside me. Even my husband fails to notice the sadness I feel when we make love because I know that our two bodies can never create a child. I feel the need to talk about it. I must tell someone this intimate fact of my life, yet I can't.

Surrogate Parenting

Choosing to have your child with the aid of a woman acting as surrogate mother is the most controversial of the now-available alternatives to traditional childbearing. The name itself conjures scientific images of labs, experiments, and robots rather than images of loving women, made of flesh and blood, bearing much-wanted babies for other couples. The adverse publicity given to several sensationalized cases belies the fact that every year dozens of couples successfully create their families through the use of surrogacy.

A couple chooses surrogacy usually because the woman is unable to carry their baby. In order to retain half of the genetic attachment to their child, they search for a willing, fertile woman to be inseminated with the man's sperm, carry the child, and give it birth. The child is adopted by the woman, or both partners jointly adopt the child, depending on the state laws.

Surrogacy is the flip side of sperm donation; the surrogate donates her egg and gestates it. It may sound simple in definition, but surrogacy is tremendously complex legally, emotionally, and ethically. Surrogacy is layered in questions, like an onion—every answered question seems to invite more questions to be asked. Any couple hoping to turn to this alternative should spend a good amount of time devoting work and thought to this method. They must decide if they are suited to it, and if they have the time, energy, emotional stability, and money to see that it goes smoothly.

Your relief in finding surrogacy to be a possible answer to your fertility problem should be well-tempered by some emotional troubleshooting. The importance of grieving for your jointly-conceived biological child is terribly important in this situation. You must be able to let go of this dream to be able to handle the complications surrogacy can bring to your feelings.

Each of you must consider how you'll be feeling throughout the process. Will the woman feel left out of the picture? Jealous of the pregnancy? Or will she experience it vicariously through the surrogate? Sometimes the surrogate and the adoptive mother can form intense bonds, and the birth, as a signal of the end of their relationship, can cause mixed feelings of joy and regret. Some women wish never to hear from the surrogate again, and fail to treat these women humanely in the days after the birth. Dealing now with your feelings may help you to relate better to the surrogate during and after the pregnancy. Or you may recognize in plenty of time that you want minimal contact with the surrogate. In some cases, you might realize surrogacy is not for you.

The man must also examine his feelings—toward the importance of biological fathering, toward his partner, toward the prospective surrogate. How do you feel about being the fertile one? Your yearning for a biologically attached child is being realized, but by bringing a third party into your lives. How do you feel about that? What are your feelings about this other woman? Do you think your attitude will change? Can you deal with the emotional reaction of your partner?

Couples must agree on the importance of biological attachment to the baby. This compelling reason is usually what steers people to surrogacy in the first place. Why is retaining this partial genetic attachment important? Are you agreed on your priorities? Are you ready to emotionally support each other, and possibly the woman acting as your surrogate? Can you "admit" a third party to your relationship, however temporarily this may be? Are your problem-solving skills ready to be put to use as small and large hitches appear in the proceedings?

State lawmakers and courts are struggling with the issues of surrogacy, as newspaper headlines show. Previous laws dealing with adoption, surrender of children to be adopted, waiting periods, baby-selling prohibitions, child custody, and even making contracts are being stretched to their limits to accommodate surrogacy. In some cases, new court rulings will be providing incentives to legislatures, where laws will be drafted. No one thinks surrogacy should be completely unregulated, yet it is impossible to define with any consensus how the laws should read.

When only a few surrogacy cases existed, arranged between the concerned parties themselves, these situations were considered private and escaped public scrutiny. Now that businesses have sprung up that screen prospective surrogates and attract childless couples, public concern isn't unwarranted.

Because surrogacy legally is so dicey, you must factor in much legal intervention if you want to try it. Research the laws in your state yourself, or find a lawyer experienced in family and adoption laws to help you. At least for now, leave the surrogate-arranging lawyers out of the picture until you know exactly what you wish to do.

Settling the legal questions is crucial, yet the ethical questions remain. Both of you must explore your feelings on these important (if over-publicized) issues. Talk these questions over privately, or with a trusted friend who can act as a devil's advocate. When called upon to defend your opinions, your true feelings will be clarified. These questions may seem inflammatory, but answering them will help you settle your minds about what you are doing.

THE ALTERNATIVES

- Is surrogacy "baby-selling" as some people charge? How can a father buy his own flesh and blood?
- Is surrogacy the renting of a human womb and nothing more? Do you think of a surrogate mother just as an incubator?
- Does surrogacy exploit women, or does outlawing it deny women freedom to use their bodies as they choose?
- Does surrogacy violate the bond of your relationship?
- Does surrogacy degrade the child's heritage?
- Isn't surrogacy the female version of AID?
- Why don't you adopt?
- Is surrogacy the same as organ donations?
- If you want a loving woman as your surrogate, how can such a woman give up her child?
- Does payment to the woman make surrogacy wrong?
- Does paying this woman seem like the only decent thing to do?
- How much payment is too little? Too much?
- Does the risk to her health taken by the surrogate during pregnancy and delivery seem worth it if she just surrenders the baby?
- Whose child is it? Who is a mother? Who is a father?
- Do you believe the reasons surrogates give for doing this?
- What will you tell the baby? What are the baby's rights?
- Are we doing this to serve ourselves or to serve the coming baby?

Practical cares and anxieties should be anticipated, too. Here are some more questions to try on for size yourselves, or with a devil's advocate:

- Do we have strong emotional reserves to devote to this process?
- Should we use a friend, a relative, or a stranger?
- Can we survive the months of the search for the surrogate, the inseminations, waiting for conception, going through the pregnancy, and the delivery?
- How friendly should we get with the surrogate?

- Should we meet face to face, talk on the phone, write letters?
- Can we share in the pregnancy experience without upsetting the surrogate?
- How can we ensure good prenatal care?
- What if she asks for more money?
- What can we do if she changes her mind? What should we do?
- Are we able to treat the surrogate well after the birth, and acknowledge her pain without feeling threatened?
- What if the child has a birth defect?
- What if the surrogate miscarries? Is it fair to "cancel" the contract?
- What do we tell our families, and why?
- Are we willing to keep the mother informed periodically through the years, if she so desires?

Until consensus develops on this issue, it might be wise to keep any surrogacy arrangement you may try as private as possible. Contracts are not enforceable, and payments may leave you open for legal intervention. Deciding on surrogacy can be the happiest decision of your life, or the stickiest. Interestingly, while many prominent feminists and legislators are coming out against surrogacy, the joy it can bring to childless couples isn't mentioned. If you are set on this alternative, for whatever reason you may have, going slowly, carefully, and thoughtfully is the only way.

Alternatives to the Alternatives: Of Eggs and Embryos

The science and technology of reproduction is speeding along, and new ways to help people have children continue to emerge. But it remains true that these advances have moved ahead of our society's legal, ethical, and religious codes. That's why these methods of fertility enhancement are so controversial.

The sensationalism that surrounds these new methods clouds the fact that as yet few couples can obtain them. The large medical teaching and research centers usually are the trailblazers, and these facilities just aren't available to everyone. Plus, the techniques are not perfected, and failure rates are quite high. Some observers feel these advances are the result of pure research being carried out on unwitting infertile women—for a fee. These critics don't understand the pain and desperation of infertility, and how willing the procedures' participants can be. Each of us must decide how we feel as the list of alternatives continues to expand.

Embryo Transfer

If a woman cannot produce an egg, but could carry a baby to term, embryo transfer may be the answer. This process involves another woman who will volunteer to donate her egg and provide her body as the fertilization site for the egg. After artificial insemination has successfully led to conception, doctors flush the embryo from the donor's body, and transfer it to the uterus of the "adoptive" mother. If the cycles of the two women are carefully synchronized, and if luck holds, the baby can be carried to term. She has given birth to her partner's biological child, but is not genetically attached to it herself.

The ethical questions involved here are many. They include the issue of payments to the donor. Should the volunteer be paid at all? Don't the physical risk involved, the nuisance of taking fertility drugs, and undergoing the transfer procedure call for any compensation? Would a woman do this otherwise?

The fate of the embryo also must be addressed. What if the fertilized egg is lost? Was a potential human life wasted? Who is the mother of this embryo? What if the embryo can't be flushed out, and becomes an unwanted pregnancy for the volunteer? What if the receiving woman's cycle doesn't respond to the regulation of fertility drugs, and she cannot take the embryo? What happens to extra embryos that are not transferred?

This technique could be the answer for couples who feel they have no choice but to search for a surrogate mother for their child. The volunteer woman in embryo transfer remains anonymous, plus the obvious pregnancy of the "once infertile" woman makes this method easier to keep discreetly quiet. It is probably less emotionally wrenching for the volunteer than carrying a baby to term. If all three participants have carefully considered their actions, the situation presents a way for a couple to participate in the creation of their baby more fully than was possible before. But there are many ethical questions involved here, so celebrating this alternative may be premature at this point.

Egg Donation

This is a less complex variation of embryo transfer. A woman undergoing IVF or even a woman facing hysterectomy or tubal ligation can elect to donate her unwanted, unused eggs. They can be harvested, fertilized in vitro, and transferred to the uterus of another woman.

The woman volunteering her eggs must be treated with fertility drugs, and her eggs are obtained during her other, previously scheduled surgical procedure. The risks of using fertility drugs and undergoing extra medical and surgical procedures are minimally compensated in some cases, but no doctor has thus far defined this practice as "buying" eggs from women.

Egg donation has been termed as the most similar counterpart of sperm donation in men. It is handled anonymously, and the volunteer woman is not even told if her donated egg is successfully fertilized and transferred.

Ethical questions do remain, however, such as the questions surrounding payment to the volunteer for her risk and trouble. (Sperm donation is infinitely simpler.) Could adequate compensation and higher success rates cause this to grow into a cottage industry? The demand will certainly be there for egg donation when medical progress brings the success rate up, but will social attitudes be able to adjust?

Embryo Freezing

Women in IVF programs can produce more than the necessary number of eggs when their ovaries are stimulated by fertility drugs. Doctors can harvest them all, fertilize them all, transfer some to the uterus immediately, and freeze the rest. The embryos are thawed and used for subsequent attempts. Theoretically, the woman is saved the rigors of taking fertility drugs later, and has insurance if she stops producing eggs or her partner stops producing good sperm for fertilization. The woman who can produce eggs can use all of them, even if not all in one cycle. An odd side effect of embryo freezing is that the number of eggs donated to other women has gone down.

Freezing is not a sure thing. Many embryos do not survive intact. If you are considering freezing your extra embryos produced during an IVF attempt, think about how you feel about freezing and thawing a potential human life, and its risk of being lost. Questions about "orphan embryos" have already come up, should the embryo survive the parents. You must decide if you feel these techniques constitute real help for infertility or if they are medical experimentation.

These newest infertility fighting techniques are, of course, trying to help couples who face one of the sadder and more painful of human situations—the inability to easily conceive and bear a child. But too often these alternatives ignore the humanity of the patients and potential children involved, and we are left confused and unsure of what is right and reasonable. Those who orchestrate these advances, as well as we the prospective patients, must always keep in mind our moral bearings as we rush into the future

Deciding to End Medical Treatment

The decision to stop medical treatment for infertility may at first glance seem to be the very opposite of what you've been striving for. But after months or years of tests, medication, surgery, and timed sex, walking away from treatment might be the right thing to do—if you're ready to do it.

Only you can tell at what point you've had enough. Your doctors can try to subtly guide you, but since infertility treatment is elective, you must make the final decision yourselves. Listen to your gut feelings and try to keep in mind your plan for treatment. How well is the timetable working out? Are you closer to your goals? Are you still within the "window of opportunity" after your surgery? How is your body holding up? How is your quality of life? Your relationship? How are your finances holding out?

Everybody has a different limit. Some couples start planning for alternatives fairly early on in medical treatment and when they reach their limits, they are prepared to try something else. Others have strength reserves to continue for quite a while, still feeling fine. Others may keep going to a point beyond their limits, and sometimes even beyond the safety of their own health. Most of us do have the inner voice that says, "Enough." But it takes courage to recognize this voice and heed it.

When we get close to our limits, we begin to notice lots of negatives connected with the medical treatments and the timed-sex routine. The negatives were once far outstripped by one positive—the chance to have a biological baby. But now the negatives weigh heavily. Watch for some of these factors cropping up in your life:

- Do you and your spouse feel tired constantly, both physically and emotionally? Are you feeling worn out all the time?
- Do you feel sad or depressed much more than you used to, but for no big or new reason?
- Are you finding it harder to be optimistic about your next cycle or treatment?
- Do you glumly anticipate a treatment's failure in order to fend off disappointment?
- Are you finding it harder to follow the doctor's instructions?
- Is your physical or mental condition starting to interfere with your job?
- Has your intimate relationship started to deteriorate even further?

- Have you dropped out of your normal life for so long that you're starting to long for it again?
- Are you fighting more? A lot more?
- Do you find yourself wondering why in the world you're doing this?

There are positive reasons to consider ending treatment, too. You don't have to wait until you feel like you're falling apart before you sense it's time to move on. For example:

- Are you beginning to focus more on the child, but not the genetics of the child?
- Does the idea of stopping seem like a relief to a lot of your troubles?
- Are you redirecting your attention to other parts of your life, and drifting away from the infertility obsession?
- Have you suddenly noticed that your partner is suffering, and you want to alleviate it somehow? Would stopping help?
- Have you realized that you are a good and worthy person apart from this struggle?
- Do you feel proud of how hard you tried, but you don't need to do any more?
- Is your curiosity about nonmedical alternatives increasing?

If you are picking up on some of these signals, you don't have to stop this month, next month, or even in the very near future. But you might want to readjust your mid- to long-range plans as you see these factors playing a larger part in your life. You can gradually put on the brakes by saying, for example, "We'll give IVF four tries," and feel good about your honest efforts. Or you can get onto adoption waiting lists in the meantime, while you wind down. Talk to your doctor about what you are planning, and you'll get help bringing things to a close by giving it one last, earnest try. (Your doctor might be tired, too.)

Instead of stopping for good, you might just need a break from trying for a while. Getting away for a trial run off the treatment routine could recharge your batteries and put things into perspective. You could bounce back, raring for more, or it could show you that yes, indeed, it was time to quit. Don't be afraid of this feeling. Don't feel guilty or ashamed. You can't walk away from your honest emotions, no matter what they are. Finding out how you really feel is an accomplishment in itself.

The Relief from the Burden Was Palpable

KATIE GEORGE

We had been to three doctors for me, and two for my husband. We had each had an operation under general anesthesia. We had each taken several kinds of pills. We had been trying for four years. I guess we were just worn out.

I didn't realize how worn out I was until we tried AIH—artificial insemination, using sperm from my husband. The first insemination fell on the day of a blizzard, of course. I didn't really know how to bring the semen in to the doctor's, so my husband just deposited it into a glass jar, like we did for his semen analyses. When I got to the doctor's office, they told me that this wouldn't do—why didn't I keep the semen at skin temperature? I didn't know I had to. The doctor insisted he had told my husband what to do. My husband later swore the doctor didn't mention it. Needless to say, I didn't enjoy being in the middle, and I was nervous enough about the insemination!

This was not a terrific way to begin a new treatment for infertility. The doctor told me that the semen I brought in was of very poor quality because it was kept too cold for too long. He said he'd inseminate me anyway, on the outside chance that some of the sperm were still OK. I glumly agreed, but I felt pretty fatalistic about it.

My temperature did not go up, and I returned for another insemination two days later. This time the doctor wasn't there—an assistant I didn't know would do the insemination instead. I felt funny that I hadn't known that others would inseminate me. Was I wrong to think this is a delicate and personal thing?

The assistant told me that again the sperm I'd brought is was of poor quality for much chance of success. Of course the sperm quality is bad, I thought: that's why we need artificial insemination! I had tried this time to keep it warm, but it wasn't all that great to start with. I was really getting depressed by this time.

As I left the doctor's office, I already sensed that this had been my last medical experience directly connected to our infertility. I had had enough. I knew that next month we were to try sperm washing, and that we could even try donor insemination eventually, or turn to IVF or GIFT. The thing was, I couldn't imagine going through with any of those treatments anymore. My strength was gone. It was time to get off the merry-go-round.

We had been going to a counselor, and he helped us realize that our life was being gobbled up by our tries for a pregnancy. He gently told us that we had a right to decide when and if we wanted to stop medical intervention. By this time the idea of stopping was like finding an oasis in the desert. We needed renewal and refreshment, and we needed to stop and rest, too.

Though I now knew that I wanted to stop, it was still hard. I realized that this was a big step, and that this decision rested upon our shoulders alone. No doctor would insist we stop. And, it looked like our bodies would not decide for us by making me pregnant without going through more hell. We just couldn't pass the buck. We had to say it.

I felt as though I was pulling the plug on a patient being maintained on a respirator. Yes, the patient is alive, but in a state of suspended animation from which he may never return. There's always a chance if you keep trying, but. . . was this the way we wanted to keep on living, for an indefinite period of time? I realized that it was not.

Deciding to quit gave me mixed feelings of guilt and relief. Why couldn't we do more? Specifically, why wasn't I strong enough to keep going on and on? I knew that some people do keep on trying and trying, and I felt badly that I just could not. But the relief from the burden was palpable. A great deal of anxiety drained out of me almost immediately. That's how I knew that it was the right thing to do.

There were advantages to stopping. I finally was freed from that nagging feeling that I was a sick patient, constantly running to the doctor for help. Four years of it had really gotten me down. I had come to think of myself as defective. Getting away from the medical treatments allowed me to start becoming a whole person again.

My husband and I also got out of the rut of having to make love at certain important times of the month, and I know he was glad that he'd never have to go through sperm analysis again. I had long feared that we would bankrupt ourselves if we needed any more operations, and suddenly our financial woes were lessened, too.

But how would we know stopping was the right thing to do—five years from now? This worry did trouble me. I thought about the relief I felt when we talked about quitting, and that helped tell me it was right. But the real sign was when it was proposed, about a year later, that we start trying again. A panic shot through me like a current of electricity. That's when I knew that what we were doing was absolutely the right thing. I was finished with that part of my life—for once and for all.

Now what do we do? We're talking about adopting, and we're even talking about what our life would be like if we don't adopt, too. It's hard, and it's scary, but we are doing it.

We are at peace with our decision to stop medical care for infertility. It wasn't easy to make. My girlfriend and my neighbor both got pregnant recently, and that hasn't helped. But deep inside I still know that the course of action we picked was best for us.

Adoption

You don't have to be superhuman, superkind, superloving, or perfect to be able to adopt a child—you just have to be ready.

Being ready only happens when you've had time to get used to the idea. This can happen suddenly or gradually, but not before you've been able to think about your personal situation, and to realistically assess your chances of having a biological or partially attached biological child.

The Earliest Questions You Have About Adoption

You begin to ask yourselves an important question: can we love an adopted child as our own? To couples just beginning to consider adoption, this is a central question, and it can be a scary one. Other preliminary questions or doubts that you may have include:

- What kind of children are available for adoption? Aren't they all misfits in one way or another?
- How could we withstand the pressure of the home study, where a social worker or other adoption authority comes into our home and judges us?

- How can we turn over this much control to other people (adoption workers) who don't even know us?
- Won't adopted children grow up maladjusted?
- Are adopted children our real children?
- What will our families say and do? Will they love a child we adopt?
- Even if we want to adopt, the wait will kill us.
- Independent adoption sounds like baby selling. Is it?
- If we're not perfect no agency will accept us anyway.
- I can't believe we have to adopt children of another nationality or race in order to obtain a child.
- Are we bad people because we'd like a baby the same race as we are, and who is normal and healthy?
- Kids are the same the whole world over, aren't they? Would an internationally adopted child feel like ours?
- Do we have to take a "waiting" or "special" child even though we are unsure?
- Won't the child go off to find its birth parents anyway?
- Why do we have to go through so much agony to build a family? Infertility was one struggle, now adoption is a whole new one.

As you find yourselves more ready to accept adoption as an alternative, these questions often lose their importance. You can let some of them go by grieving for your biological child. Others disappear after you do some talking with adoptive parents, watching adoption-built families together, reading books on adoption, and learning how adoption is really accomplished.

The process of grieving for your biological child is an important step in becoming ready to consider adoption. A couple must, together and separately, come to terms with their loss. They must go through the stages of denial, anger, and depression, along with their urges to atone or bargain to deserve a child. You gradually learn to say good-bye.

Until you have grieved, adoption may not attract you. The adoptable kids will not appeal to you, and the trouble it takes to adopt will not seem worth it. Through grief, you learn to focus less on the process of obtaining children and more on the children themselves. As you grieve, you must ask yourself what your parenting goals really are.

For women, a goal to be reconsidered is that of pregnancy, of giving birth and breastfeeding. These experiences can be central to a woman's desired identity, and she may need a biological child in order to feel fulfilled. But ask yourself what a mother really is. Is it nine months of gestating, or is it twenty years of nurturing? Only you can say what is of primary importance to you. If you can gradually let go of this dream and think about the child itself, you could be suited to adoption.

If you both have grieved you will be free to choose or not choose adoption, and you won't feel forced by adverse circumstances or bad luck. If you reject adoption after grieving, you can know that you made this choice not as a rejection out of anger, frustration, or depression. You will be free to realize that it's just not right for you, and that that's OK, too.

If you move toward acceptance of adoption as an alternative suited to you, you begin to change your focus, and the importance of blood ties diminishes. The amount of time adoption takes, the form of adoption that's right for you, how to do it, and worries about what may go wrong now come into play. The question is no longer, "Can we do this?" but becomes, "How do we do this?"

Trying on adoption in your imaginations helps make it a real possibility, not a remote and abstract concept. When you think about adoption and how it could come into your life, you must have the correct information. Basing your mind's pictures on myths won't do you any good at all. Learning about adoption becomes your first job.

READ. There are many books and publications available on adoption. Many are specialized to a single method of adoption, such as international, special-needs, traditional agency-oriented. You can send for the newsletters of adoptive parents' organizations, national support groups, placement advocates. Ask to be put on their mailing lists. You can read over all the paperwork of a friend who has adopted. Send for RESOLVE's information on adoption—they have a lot, too. Go over whatever you can find, and mull it over. You'll learn a lot, and you can keep your privacy, if you need it now.

TALK. Talk to adoptive parents you may know, to members of a local adoptive parents' organization, to agency representatives, to adopted kids themselves. Find out what it's like to adopt from a personal viewpoint. Find out that adopted kids do just fine by meeting some.

ASK. Ask any and all of your questions. Call for information. Call agencies, lawyers, organizations, a RESOLVE contact person. Remain anonymous on the phone if you like. But you need to have your questions put to rest before you can accept adoption fully, so try and get your answers as best you can.

NETWORK. This is a natural offshoot of talking and asking. If you know someone who knows someone who adopted in a way that interests you, networking gets you to that person. Ask around. Adoptive parents are almost to a person eager to help others with their questions. You could turn up some pretty interesting tips on what to do and how to cope. Go to a preliminary meeting of an adoptive parents' organization or support group. What you hear may just get you started.

Types of Adoption

Agency Adoption Traditional, agency-assisted adoption was once the common way to adopt kids. Due to a variety of factors, this is no longer the case. Experts blame abortion and the changing of societal stigmas against unwed motherhood as two big reasons. Whatever the explanation, agency adoption of healthy white infants is still possible, but usually takes a very long time. The adoption procedure moves more quickly for black parents adopting healthy black children through agencies than domestic trans-racial adoptions do. Agencies are sometimes accused of being too picky because they place so few children. And many infertile couples find that waiting so long for a biological child has made waiting a long period again for an agency-placed child very difficult.

Research, by relentlessly calling agencies on the phone, can uncover agencies with shorter waits or the requirements that you can live with. But whatever agency you go with, be prepared to feel a loss of some control. It simply goes with the territory. Adoption workers are individuals, and should not be lumped together, but because they are seen by you to have the power to "grant" you your wish (a child), you may view them as formidable.

In many states, and with most agencies, investigating you is required before you qualify to adopt. It may include a questionnaire, interviews, giving references, scrutiny of your employment circumstances, visits to your home. You may feel you are being judged, and you may feel resentment. This doesn't make you bad—it makes you normal. But try to see it from the agency's point of view. How can they find out about you without asking questions? Should they simply give you a baby just because you asked? Of course not. So resign yourselves to make it through your home study with a realistic attitude.

Agency adoption can be time consuming, but it offers valuable services: first, you do not have to search out birth parents who are ready to give up their unwanted child. Next, you are assured that all legal requirements are being observed. And you can be sure the child has been surrendered and that it is yours. Being free of these worries can be most important considerations for some couples, and make the waiting and scrutiny worthwhile.

International Adoption International adoption is an alternative that is growing in popularity, thanks largely to a handful of "adopter-friendly" countries such as Korea, Columbia, Chile, and India. There are agencies that are specially devoted to handling international adoptions. They investigate and do home studies like traditional agencies, but the wait for an international child is almost always much shorter. There is lots of paperwork with international adoptions, and the baby has to become an American citizen. Sometimes there is bureaucratic red tape to cut through. The cost is not low. In some cases you may be required to travel abroad to pick up your child.

Adopting a child of another nationality isn't done only by "bleeding hearts" or superhumans. Regular people just like you can discover how easy it is to love an adopted child, international kids included. There may be some additional considerations you should make, though. You may need to reassure yourselves that you can help your child fit in comfortably in his new home, neighborhood, school, town. Also, you should allow your families to get used to the idea of international adoption. You do not need their approval, but having their support can be important. Give them information and any other help they need. You needed help with this once, too, and they will come around as you did.

Support groups for parents adopting international kids can assist you. You will pick up lots of stories and advice on how to make your child feel absolutely at home with you, yet cherish his native culture if he chooses.

Independent Adoption The next type of adoption actually has three different names. Independent adoption, private adoption, and identified adoption all refer to the adopting of children found through your own initiative. This requires lots of work, research, problem-solving skills, suspense, risk of disappointment, and legal assistance. In some states (check your local laws) it also frees you from the investigations of a home study. Adopting independently can be a breeze or it can be a very rocky road. Usually it is somewhere in between.

You, or a representative you designate, must start searching for a pregnant woman who is planning to give up her child for adoption. Remember, you are looking for someone who has already made this decision, so you aren't coercing anyone. There are various methods for conducting this search, and some may be more acceptable to you than others. Placing newspaper ads (where legal), reaching ob-gyns, or using a "resumé" that goes to a child-search agency are all methods that have worked. Find out many more by talking to parents who have independently adopted. Go to meetings of adoptive parents and ask around. You'll be amazed and encouraged by the stories that you hear. What you learn through this kind of networking you'll not find in adoption books, no matter how complete. You'll not only learn what to do, but you'll be warned about what not to do. That information is equally valuable.

There is emotional and financial risk to independent adoption. The birth mother could change her mind during the pregnancy, or right after the birth. In some states there is a lengthy waiting period before the official surrender of custody, and you could find this wait very difficult. The birth mother may ask for support and expenses during her pregnancy, which most independent adopters do pay. But be careful: ask your lawyer about all the legal angles of independent adoption before you start the entire process, and especially before you make any payments. There is also a risk that the baby's biological father may make his wishes known, which may not agree with the birth mother's. In many cases, you can talk with or meet the birth mother. Some women form an intense relationship with the birth mother of their coming adopted child. This could make your situation easier or more complicated.

Don't believe all the sensationalized stories about independent adoption. It is legal. It isn't baby selling. It isn't coercion. You can only get the whole picture by researching the legal aspects with a qualified adoption lawyer and asking adoptive parents. With this method you can adopt a healthy infant of your race in a shorter period of time than if you wait for an agency's help. This is the biggest advantage of independent adoption, and can make all the hassles worthwhile.

Special Needs Kids   Waiting children, or special-needs kids, are adoptable children who are older, of mixed racial heritage, are handicapped, or are in sibling groups. Because they are harder to place, the wait for them is sometimes shorter. This doesn't mean, however, that an agency will speed up the adoption process for an infertile couple with no other adopted children.

You shouldn't consider adopting special-needs kids unless you want them for their own qualities. Don't view them as "all we can get." Don't take on the task of raising them only to atone for past sins. Don't feel you have to want them just because they are available. If you want a healthy infant of your own race, don't feel guilty about this. If special-needs kids aren't for you, you shouldn't consider adopting them for the wrong reasons.

But if you really want to adopt this way, be persistent. Adoption workers may try to screen you out. If you are eager to take special-needs kids into your hearts and your home, this message will eventually get through if you are diligent and do not give up. A well-considered decision to adopt special-needs kids requires even more networking, talking, asking, and reading so that you can discover your capabilities. Do your homework, ask your heart, then make up your minds.

Some Facts of Life About Adoption

Adoption does not "cure" infertility. There's a big myth floating around that in order to become pregnant, you should adopt first. In fact, there is no cause-and-effect relationship here. Adopted children with younger biological siblings are common, but they are the result of completely independent factors. There are even more adopted kids with no biological siblings.

Adoption doesn't cure the physical aspects of infertility, nor does it cure the emotional pain of infertility. Bringing an adopted child into your home will not instantly erase the months or years of infertility and the effect infertility has had on your emotions. You will still feel a twinge of sadness now and then, but it will gradually recede on its own. Having a child in the house naturally takes the center of attention away from your past problems, which can only help. But infertility and adoption are separate entities.

By the same token, don't worry that every time you look at this child, you will be reminded that you are infertile. This doesn't happen. If you have grieved and let go, your child will be your child, no matter how you came to have him. If you find this hard to accept, you may not yet be ready to take the step of adoption. Give yourself more time to grieve.

Adoption may be your second choice, but it's just as good as biological parenting. Don't try to compare them. They're different, and one isn't better than the other. Recalling your special telephone call announcing the birth or arrival of your child is just as precious a memory as that of labor and birth.

Adoption is a lot of work. A baby isn't going to fall into your lap. No matter which type of adoption you choose it will involve paperwork, asking questions, spending money, emotional ups and downs, interpersonal skills, problem solving, researching, risk. Those who want to adopt will always succeed. But it takes time and work. It is unfair that most biological parents will never know how much you went through, but it remains a fact that this work will be required of you. Adoptive parent support groups exist to help you every step of the way, and they do understand how difficult it can be. But they can also testify that yes, the work will pay off, and you will be parents.

As you consider adoption, realize that your feelings may change over time. As you get more used to the idea of adoption and learn about it, your misconceptions will give way to a realistic attitude. Each of you must grapple with adoption separately, then come to a decision together. First, bat around your feelings and ideas in a nonthreatening atmosphere. At first, adoption can be a touchy subject, and feelings may run high. Each of you is entitled to your opinion—just be sure it is based on truths.

Even if one or both of you is unsure about adoption, you may be able to sense that your opinion will move in a more positive direction with time. You may feel that you're on the way, but you're just not there yet. You need more time to work it out. But if time is a precious commodity for you, you might have to make some arrangements in advance.

You can go ahead and place your names on agencies' waiting lists. In cases where there are long waits, you shouldn't hold off until you are absolutely positive before you even pick up the phone. Later on, when your name gets to the top of an agency list and you are called for an intake interview, you will probably know your mind. You can accept the appointment, or you can turn it down and give your place to someone else. It's your choice, but you haven't wasted any time.

Are You Ready to Be a Mom?

MARY MASON

*O*n February 25, at 6:05 P.M., the phone rang. When I answered I heard my social worker from the Children's Home Society ask me, "Mary, are you ready to be a mom?" At 1:00 P.M. the following day we were to pick up our three-and-a-half-week-old son.

Was I ready to be a mom? I wanted to scream the answer into the phone, to paint it on the curb, to hire a skywriter. Ready? I was about six and a half years beyond ready. After Doug and I married in 1979, we immediately tried to get pregnant. I trotted off to the doctor for a rubella test, since I was adopted at age two and no one had my early medical records. The medical staff was so pleasant, so full of optimism when the test came back negative. It was the beginning of many negative tests, years of charting, microsurgery, an entourage of doctors who would make the staff of "St. Elsewhere" look like bit players, and of constantly watching Doug on the opposite end of the seesaw of emotions.

Halfway through this ongoing crisis I found RESOLVE. As with anything in life that I care about, I became consumed with the group. It has become a very positive consumption, because by serving this organization, I have been able to work out frustration after frustration in a constructive way. I have selfishly tapped into the latest information on medical, emotional aspects of infertility, and the options available. When my final medical prognosis was dismal, RESOLVE members bolstered me. When the state adoption statistics I heard were discouraging, I remembered through RESOLVE to be persistent. It worked for us with a wonderful result: Joshua Robert.

The evening of that fateful phone call, I had to open the RESOLVE meeting. The topic that evening—adoption. Those who attended the meeting heard my voice break as I shared the news, and it was very special to me that everyone immediately applauded. That's how it feels to adopt. You want to applaud yourself, and everyone around you is applauding, too. I'm amazed at the outpouring of support we've received as we've received Joshua, not just from those who understand how much it means to finally have a child, but from the fertile world. It's as if they were always there but simply didn't know how to express their concern.

Despite the miracle of little Josh, I am reminded from time to time of my infertility. I am reminded because his birth mother also named him Joshua. I am reminded when a stranger asks me how my pregnancy went and a woman at a baby shower exclaims, "But he's so perfect. What was wrong with his mother that she gave him up?" Sometimes the reminder is pleasant, as when my mother-in-law wanted us to be sure to tell the pediatrician of the diabetes in our family. I know now that Grandma considers Josh as much her blood as we do.

These past years have been an incredible journey, not always painful, not always joyous, but always full of growth. I give much credit and loyalty to RESOLVE for teaching me that infertility can offer resolution for those who persistently work through it. I can enjoy my son now not because my infertility is over, but because I am comfortable with it. Am I ready to be a mom? Yes, resoundingly, yes.

(Mary Mason has been president of the Twin Cities RESOLVE. She is the author of The Miracle Seekers, *a book of short stories about infertility, published by Perspectives Press.)*

Childfree Living

To live happily without children after struggling with infertility—does it sound unthinkable, impossible, crazy, pathetic? If this decision is right for you, living childfree is none of these things. It marks the end of your battle against infertility, but it is not a defeat if your decision is freely and carefully considered.

Why the word "childfree" instead of "childless"? This unfamiliar term may sound like jargon to you now, but using "childfree" implies a positive, happy release from the trap of infertility, while "childless" is a negative word implying a loss. Living childfree is a legitimate path you can choose, not just a case of settling for misery forever.

Arriving at the childfree decision isn't a piece of cake. It requires grieving, soul searching, absolutely frank communication with your partner, and a search for renewed commitment together. It means facing a part of yourself that at first you may not want to meet. It means accepting your deepest feelings without fighting them. It can mean risking the misunderstanding of others around you. But for the right people, it brings resolution to infertility in a way no other alternative can.

How can this decision emerge as a possibility when all this time you've been preoccupied with having children? It happens gradually as you find your goals changing, your attitudes toward infertility changing, your self-image changing. Your fundamental wishes and desires start to reveal themselves. and you reach a point where you can recognize them.

Sometimes the desire and need to create a child together privately, naturally, and with love is all a couple has ever wanted. Months or years of infertility and medical intervention can rob them of this joyful opportunity, leaving them unsettled and dissatisfied. They can lose their desire for medical intervention and simply find they've run out of energy.

In other cases, alternatives become impossible or inappropriate for personal or medical reasons, and childfree life becomes a threat that must be grappled with. Once a couple faces what childfree living actually is, it may lose its negative connotations and become a positive way to resolve infertility.

Couples may find that their motives change over time, or that they each may be coping with their infertility in different ways. Childfree living can become a temporary or permanent compromise worth considering.

Remember, no one alternative to natural, total biological parenting is suitable to everybody. That's why there are so many to choose from. Each alternative meets certain needs. It may seem odd to think that a childfree decision can actually meet your needs, but for the right people, it certainly does.

- **Childfree living fills** the need to get on with life in a positive way. After months or years of sadness, setbacks, and disappointments, couples can have a very depressing, negative attitude towards themselves and one another. They may realize one day that their entire outlook on life has been warped by infertility, making all things look bleak. It becomes impossible to wait around any longer for a baby to make them happy again. Childfree living becomes a positive, necessary, and lifesaving decision they can make.

- **Childfree living meets** the need for a temporary compromise while couples attempt to become "synchronized" in their decision making. If one partner just cannot accept adoption yet, for example, an agreement to remain childfree in the interim may work.

  The decision can become a permanent, positive one even if it originally was made for a compromise. If it becomes clear that compromise or agreement may never come, disagreeing couples leave their choices behind and approach childfree living positively, together. It is extremely difficult, but it can be done. Sometimes this is the only way to save a relationship.

- **This decision can** bring a feeling of peace, acceptance, and even spirituality that no other alternative can bring. A couple has decided together to forego something they wanted very much. Now they can turn outward, to enrich their own lives and the lives of those around them in their families and communities. Childfree living is an acceptance, not a sacrifice.

- **Through the months** or years of treatment, couples can lose sight of their original goal: having a baby. The struggle to overcome infertility can be so overwhelming, it can blot out this goal. One day, couples may just wake up and say, "What is all this for, anyhow??" Realizing that the battle has been against the doctor, against powerlessness, or simply as a way to vent rage is a step toward recognition of the childfree alternative. If the baby has disappeared from your thoughts for months at a time but you are still grimly determined to succeed with treatments, perhaps your goals have shifted. Considering childfree living might be a nonthreatening way to begin to accept that children aren't your goal anymore.

- **A carefully thought** out childfree decision can quickly bring peace into your life. Months or years of uncertainty are now over. You don't have to face any more doctors, medical procedures, medication, adoption workers, lawyers. There are no more hurdles to moving toward your new life.
- **Childfree living is** an opportunity to build a marital relationship that is special, rich, and deep. You can focus on one another freely and happily, maybe for the first time in years. As much as you longed for a child, it's a fact that couples with children must work extra hard to keep their relationship as it once was. You can be proud that you are a family together, unto yourselves—you don't need a child to make it official.
- **Childfree life affords** freedom to pursue both individual and joint interests and gives you more time to work hard in your careers. It lends a unique perspective to the value of time and its use. If you plan your new life positively and energetically, the pursuit of productivity in areas other than in child-rearing will help new, deep fulfillments begin to grow.

Just as with all the other alternatives, considering childfree living doesn't mean you have to do it. Presenting it as an option isn't going to change or threaten your true feelings. On the contrary, it will help you to find them. So don't be afraid to try it on for size. You should each think carefully about your individual feelings regarding parenthood. Then together you can discuss your thoughts and begin to approach a decision when you're ready. Give yourselves lots of time. Play devil's advocate with some of these questions:

- What are your motives now for having a child? Do you remember what they were when you first started trying? Are these motives now different?
- Are you so tired that you'd just like to take a break? Or are you afraid you really want to walk away from all this for good? Why does that scare you?
- What kind of energy do you have left to pursue complex alternatives? Does tackling these alternatives appeal to you? Or do you just feel that after coming this far, you ought to do something, anything?
- What are your biggest fears about remaining childfree? Are they logical, emotional, or somewhere in between? When you say them out loud do they sound like sense or nonsense? Ask yourselves, "What is

the worst thing that could happen if we remain childfree? We'll be alone in old age? I'll be alone if my spouse dies? Our marriage will have no meaning? We'll look different to our family and friends? People will feel sorry for us? People will think we're quitters? People will think we hate kids? We'll miss out on a major life experience? We wanted the chance to nurture our own child, and we'll miss that? Nobody will call us Mommy and Daddy? How would we fill our life? We'll have to shape a different life than what we planned? We won't ever feel grown up? Our parents won't love us like they would if we give them grandchildren? We won't live on through our children; mortality seems so near? We're afraid that remaining childfree may mean that we never wanted children in the first place?"

Infertility cuts through pretense. It clarifies values. Couples dealing with it must confront their feelings, goals, their phobias, neuroses, and hang-ups as they struggle to find resolution. It can make you see life in an entirely new context. Facing basic truths about yourselves and one another is scary, because you're dealing with issues you'd probably rather avoid. But if you have had the courage to do this, the freedom from the burden of pretense is exhilarating.

Couples who choose positively to become childfree have probably discovered these things about themselves:

- That we have lost sight of the child for its own sake. We were doing battle with forces larger than ourselves. This struggle is no longer about a child, and we see this now. Realizing this does not make us bad people.

- We are not the kind of people who would do just anything in order to get a child. We have our limits, which we are not ashamed of. We are glad that we have been able to identify these limits and accept them.

- The quality of our relationship is highly important to us. Our life is deteriorating due to this struggle, to the point where even finally getting a child may not improve it. We want to stop and work on our commitment.

- We have what looks like a lasting disagreement about what course of action is best for us. We are each entitled to our feelings. Because we cannot agree but still love one another, childfree life is our best compromise.

- All we originally wanted was our biological child, conceived the old-fashioned way. There is nothing wrong with this goal, but because this was our goal alone, alternatives would not be satisfying.
- We don't feel right about adopting, and we are smart enough not to let societal pressure force us into a decision that isn't right for us.
- We are worthy people whether or not we choose to have children. We don't need a child just to confirm our worthiness.
- Each of us feels that our partner is our most important family member—not a child who does not yet exist, and who we may never obtain. Two can make a family and have a good life.
- We do not feel selfish about this decision. We can be proud that we found the decision that is right for us. We don't need to prove to others that we are unselfish just by battling on to find a child.

As you move toward a decision to remain childfree, you will begin to experience certain realities that come along with it, mostly in the form of societal attitudes that may clash with your choice.

A childfree choice is unusual. It will be commented upon by friends and acquaintances, even strangers if you get that far in conversation. Others may love to psychoanalyze you, and they'll come up with various theories that will please them but that will remain nonsense. People with children, especially those of your parents' generation, may press you to follow in their footsteps and confirm their life choices. They may imply that they know something you don't know. You are under no obligation to prop up other people's self-doubts with your own life! Enduring these comments will be difficult at first, when your decision is new. It will become easier to deal with in time, and you'll probably develop a couple of surefire comebacks to shut such people up. You are not obligated to explain your decision to anybody, so don't get defensive.

Even your friends who are infertile may feel threatened by your childfree choice. Realize that they may not be as "far along" in their thinking and may fear facing certain facts about themselves that your choice suggests to them. Choosing to remain childfree can be misconstrued as disapproval of their own choices, and they may become defensive. They may put you on the defensive. Remember their pain—it was your pain once—and try to understand.

As you choose childfree living, you'll wonder about the choices you leave behind. You're bound to. Nobody is ever absolutely sure all the time time that they're doing the right thing. You will be no different. Having doubts doesn't mean you've made a bad choice. If you came to this decision slowly and deliberately, you can have confidence in it.

Even as you realize this decision is correct, you'll still feel sad when you hear about the pregnancies of family and friends. Again, this doesn't mean you're wrong—it means you're human.

Remaining childfree cannot exist as a legitimate, satisfying alternative until each partner has grieved for your child. No childfree life can be lived with peace of mind until you realize, through grief, what you have lost. After grieving, you will be able to accept that other alternatives just don't suit you, and you won't confuse the rejection of those options with grief-induced rage, depression, or denial. You are free to let go of inappropriate resolutions without self-recrimination or intense doubts. You will gradually become comfortable with your newly emerging identity.

After you make this choice—nothing happens. You may not feel at first like your life has changed. Nothing earth-shattering will take place to mark your choice unless you arrange for it yourselves. When you realize this, you'll recognize the importance of inaugurating your decision with some kind of action to make it official. Some couples even have tubal ligations or vasectomies so they will never wonder "what if" again. You can change your lifestyle in a major way by going back to school, moving to a new home, beginning to reach out to others socially, or giving a helping hand. Have you considered getting married again (to each other, of course!), taking a dream vacation, throwing your first big party in ages? Think of a joyous way to seal your commitment.

Even if you do choose childfree life, you may still wonder, why did we do all this? It may be hard at times to come to terms with your infertility struggle. You may feel that you've been through a strange, meaningless trial by fire. Or you may find meaning through religious faith, or through your personal philosophy of living. It will take time. Allow for that time and don't guilt-trip yourselves.

Realize that whatever the outcome, this entire experience has been profound. It may be the deepest experience you two will ever have together, and it indeed may be far deeper than the experiences of biological parents living unexamined lives. Acknowledge the immensity of this event and you'll begin to feel a sense of release. Diminishing the experience of infertility in order to justify a childfree decision will not help you to master it.

Infertility is a grave test of your commitment to one another and to your relationship. Nowhere is this more evident than with the childfree decision. Getting through this is a victory for your strength, love, patience, communication, reasoning, perseverance. You may now see within yourselves abilities you never dreamed you had. You may have seen in your partner remarkable qualities that make you ache with love and appreciation. Meeting your own pain, and that of your partner, is an invaluable human skill.

One day you'll realize that the question constantly whirling around in your brain— "Are we ever going to get through this?"— has changed, remarkably, to an answer—"Yes, we did survive this!" Strange as it may seem, this statement itself is the resolution that you both have been searching for. And finding it is your victory.

Instead We Have Found Each Other

MARGARET M. JOHNSON

Our decision to remain childfree was not an overnight decision. It came from nine years of infertility. We went from doctor to doctor, test to test, looking for an answer. We still do not have the answer. We are a "normal" infertile couple. We could continue to go to more doctors, take more drugs, try new tests. Continue to lie to our employers about another appointment. Wait at the doctor's office while pregnant women flow in and out. Keep up the hopeful waiting, month after month, year after year.

But we want to get on with our life, to enjoy the time we have, alone together. We have learned so much over the years due to our infertility. I often wonder what we would have been like if we had been fertile.

We have become very body conscious. We know every ebb and flow of our cycles. We take great pride in our bodies, even though we are infertile.

Our marriage has become much stronger. We have grown to appreciate our solitude. We are each other's best friend. We've shared a great deal together, and that makes our relationship so special. What we had hoped for was a child to share our lives. But instead we have found each other.

Oh sure, I still avoid looking at pregnant bellies. And I ache when I see baby shoes (they're so small). But the hurt has lessened with the passage of time. I have a wonderful godson, and just being a part of his life is gratifying. I have a fantastic, understanding husband, with whom I look forward to spending the rest of my life. We are a family. And that makes my life worthwhile.

THE ALTERNATIVES

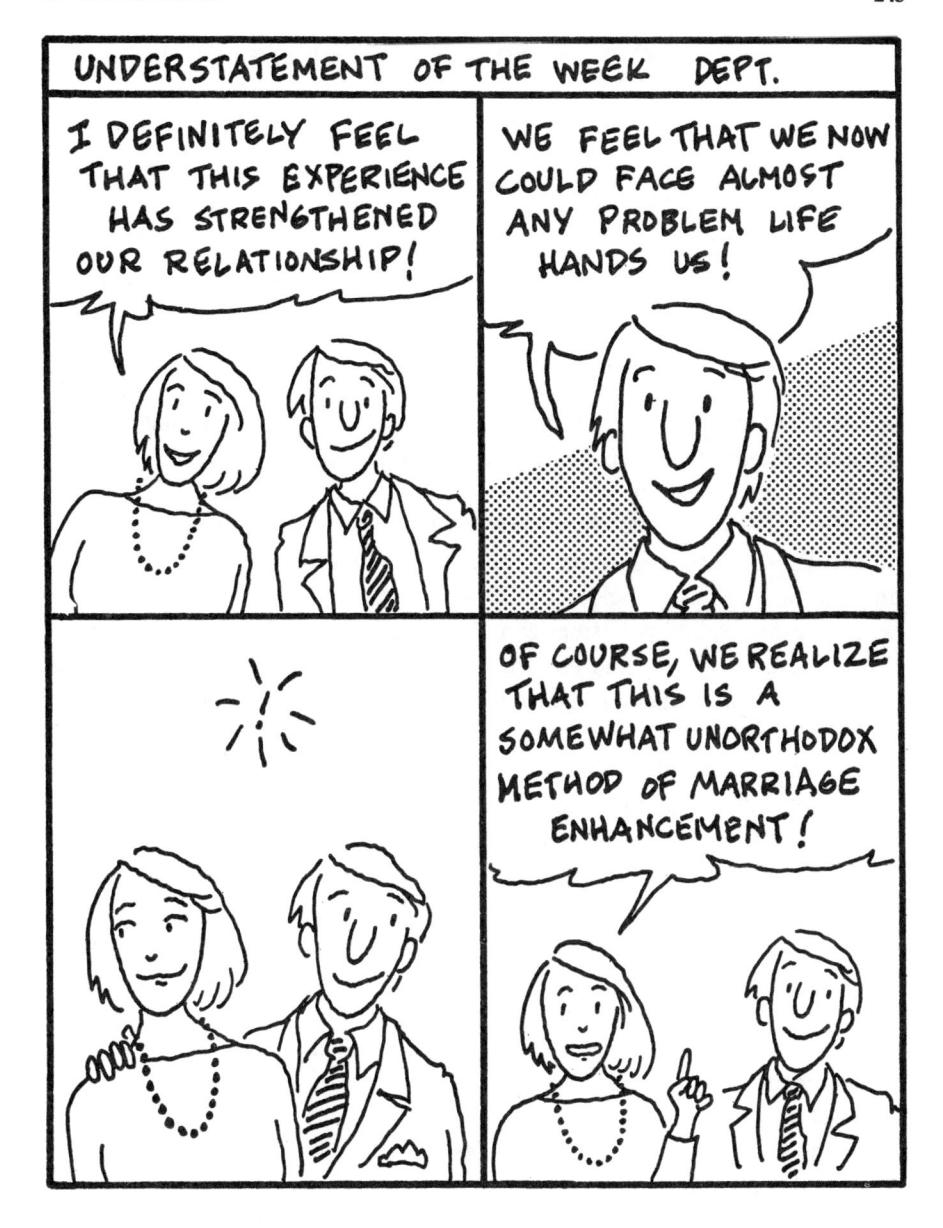

UNDERSTATEMENT OF THE WEEK DEPT.

"I DEFINITELY FEEL THAT THIS EXPERIENCE HAS STRENGTHENED OUR RELATIONSHIP!"

"WE FEEL THAT WE NOW COULD FACE ALMOST ANY PROBLEM LIFE HANDS US!"

"OF COURSE, WE REALIZE THAT THIS IS A SOMEWHAT UNORTHODOX METHOD OF MARRIAGE ENHANCEMENT!"

The Happiest Place on Earth

MARY MASON

Snowbirds from Minnesota, my husband, son, and I found ourselves in the parking lot at Disneyland. A sign lauding the amusement park as "The Happiest Place on Earth," a dangerous claim at best, greeted us. I recalled visiting Florida's Disney World years ago during a recession when hundreds of laid-off auto workers had headed south to seek the happiness that was presently eluding them. That experiment appeared not to have been working, as I witnessed screeching parents and crying children in the scorching sun.

For my husband and me, this trip to Disneyland was an odyssey of a different sort. Our son, Joshua, is the culmination of years of drugs, surgeries, and long waits in clinics and adoption agencies. Those years were full of heartache, anger, and pain so grievous we began to withdraw from the very thing we most wanted: children. That conscious choice was an effort to avoid their wonder, their fragility, their joy.

When we finally achieved a spot on an adoption agency's list, we were assured that we would receive a child. Still we relied on the old defenses, the habitual feeling of not daring to hope. But gradually we began to buy baby items, quickly darting in and out of stores. One day, when time seemed to indicate that we couldn't procrastinate any longer, we forced ourselves into the children's section of a department store. It took tremendous courage, and we felt like interlopers as we purchased a crib and a changing table.

Two weeks later our son arrived. He was a perfect fit for our lives, our family. The day after his arrival my husband turned to me and said, "It seems like he's always been with us. Can you remember what it was like before?" At that moment, I surely couldn't.

But I do remember it from time to time, like that day in Disneyland. With one in six couples affected by infertility, there had to be others like us in the crowd, even though Disneyland must be a place most infertiles might avoid for obvious reasons. In this celebrated spot for children of all ages, where strollers line up outside each attraction like shoes in Japan, I explored faces. Occasionally there would be an obvious example, like the Caucasian couple with their Korean daughter. Were there others, like us, who had planned a trip to Disneyland in celebration of a long-sought child?

Joshua became our eyes, rushing up to each Disney character like a newfound friend. He ran unencumbered down streets, with no admonition to look both ways first. Here he was encouraged to express his appreciation loudly as he encountered sights that filled his imagination: giants on stilts, motorcycle daredevils, topiary in animal shapes, matronly women and bald men wearing mouse ears.

Some might think bringing a two-year-old across a thousand miles to a glorified amusement park a bit indulgent. It is the same thinking I have encountered from the media, who ask why infertile couples go to such extremes to have a child. "What's the big deal?" their question implies.

One doesn't have to go to Disneyland to answer that question. It is through the wondering eyes of children that we renew ourselves and celebrate life. Walt Disney created his parks around that very concept.

Less and less of the world indulges or tolerates children—or even childlike ideas. On our plane to California, Joshua and two small boys played together by the bulkhead, occasionally spilling their toys into the aisle. One disgruntled man, fortified with a few drinks and on his way to the lavatory, angrily demanded to know the parents of a boy in his path. "I paid my money, too!" he bellowed. "My money is as good as anybody's." His is a voice we hear most often in the world—angry, constantly inconvenienced by the bother of innocence. That bellow stills the child's voice inside us as we madly dash towards career, status, pleasure, and, yes, children. I knew that man's voice, and his vision. It had been mine so many years ago in that other Disney World, when all I could see were angry parents and uncomfortable children. My dimmed vision could only see my own tension, and I was blind to the private celebrations around me.

It took a different trip in a different era, culminating from a different grief, to find this happiest place on earth. We were finally able to revel with other adults, all of us embracing childhood. I understand now that the happiest place on earth is not a multimillion dollar amusement park. It's not a place, a location. It lies deep inside of us, waiting to be released, if we can only discover our own innocent wonder.

Appendix

Reading up on Infertility

Here are suggestions for materials you can send for or find in libraries and bookstores. You will also find the addresses of support groups, helpful organizations, and small publishers you can write to for further information.

General Reading on Infertility

RESOLVE, Inc.
5 Water Street
Arlington, MA 02174
(617) 643-2424

Write to RESOLVE and request a listing of their fact sheets and back issues of newsletters that are available. The list is very comprehensive.

Medical Periodicals on Infertility

(find them in university or medical libraries)

- *Fertility and Sterility*
- *Contemporary Ob/Gyn*
- *Obstetrics and Gynecology*

Books: Learning About Reproduction, Fertility, and Infertility

You Can Have a Baby, by Dr. Joseph Bellina and Josleen Wilson. New York: Crown Publishers, 1985.

How to Get Pregnant, by Dr. Sherman Silber. New York: Warner Books, 1981.

Miracle Babies and Other Happy Endings, by Dr. Mark Perloe and Linda Gail Christie. New York: Rawson Associates, 1986.

Books: Readings on Specific Diagnoses, Treatments, and Alternatives

DES
Write to: DES Action National
Long Island Jewish Hospital
New Hyde Park, NY 11040

or DES Action West
2845 24th Street
San Francisco, CA 94110

Endometriosis
Write to: The Endometriosis Association
PO Box 92187
Milwaukee, WI 53202

Endometriosis, by Julia Older. New York: Charles Scribner's Sons, 1984.

Living with Endometriosis, by Kate Weinstein. Reading, Mass.: Addison-Wesley, 1987.

Overcoming Endometriosis, by Mary Lou Ballweg. Chicago: Congdon & Weed Associates, 1987.

Miscarriage
Write to: Pregnancy and Infant Loss Center
1415 E. Wayzata Blvd., Suite 22
Wayzata. MN 55391

Books:

Miscarriage: A Shattered Dream, by Sherokee Ilse. Wintergreen Press: PO Box 165, Long Lake, MN 55356.

When Pregnancy Fails: Families Coping with Miscarriage, Stillbirth, and Infant Death, by Susan Borg and Judith Lasker. Boston: The Beacon Press, 1981.

Advanced Technologies of Reproduction
New Conceptions: A Consumer's Guide to the Newest Infertility Treatments, by Lori Andrews. New York: St. Martin's Press, 1984.

Making Miracles: In-Vitro Fertilization, by Nan and Todd Hilton. New York: Doubleday, 1985.

Books: How It Feels to Be Infertile

Infertility: How Couples Can Cope, by Linda Salzer, MSW. Boston: G. K. Hall, 1986.
Infertility: A Guide for the Childless Couple, by Barbara Eck Menning. Englewood Cliffs, N.J.: Prentice-Hall, 1977; revised, 1987.
Give Us a Child, by Lynda R. Stephenson. San Francisco: Harper & Row, 1984.
The Miracle Seekers, by Mary Martin Mason. Fort Wayne, Ind.: Perspectives Press, 1987.
Understanding—A Guide to Impaired Fertility for Family and Friends, by Patricia I. Johnston. Ft. Wayne, Ind.: Perspectives Press, 1983.

Book: On Doctor/Patient Relations

Playing God: The New World of Medical Choices, by Thomas Scully, M.D., and Celia Scully. New York: Simon & Schuster, 1987.

For Listings of Specialists in Infertility, Write:
The American Fertility Society
1608 13th Ave S., Suite 101
Birmingham, AL 35205

Books: Readings for Solace or Fellowship

The Miracle Seekers, by Mary Martin Mason. Fort Wayne, Ind.: Perspectives Press, 1987.
When Bad Things Happen to Good People, by Rabbi Harold Kushner. New York: Schocken Books, 1981.
Coping with Infertility, by Judith Stigger. Minneapolis: Augsberg Publishing, 1983.

Adoption
Write to these organizations for literature and local contacts:

- OURS, Inc.
  3307 Highway 100 North, Suite 203
  Minneapolis, MN 55422

- National Adoption Exchange
  1218 Chestnut Street
  Philadelphia, PA 19107

- North American Council on Adoptable Children
  810 18th St. Suite 703
  NW Washington, DC 20006

Books:

The Adoption Resource Book, by Lois Gilman. New York: Harper & Row, 1981.

The Fifteen Most Asked Questions About Adoption, by Laura Valenti. Scottsdale, Penn.: The Herald Press, 1985. (Available through many local adoption groups.)

An Adoptor's Advocate, by Patricia Johnston. Fort Wayne, Ind.: Perspectives Press, 1984. (Perspectives Press, 905 W. Wildwood Ave., Fort Wayne, IN 46807)

Childfree Living

Books:

Childless by Choice, by Marilyn Faux. New York: Anchor Press, 1984.

The Baby Decision, by Merle Bombardieri. New York: Rawson-Wade, 1981.

Marriage Without Children, by Diana Burgwyn. New York: Harper & Row, 1982.

Insurance and Cost Recovery

Wouldn't it be great to wave your arm and say to your doctor, "Hang the cost! Do whatever it takes!"

Unfortunately, most of us cannot. No matter how badly we want a certain treatment, the high costs can make us think twice.

When in the midst of invasive testing or surgery, you can feel doubly victimized to discover the indifferent attitude most insurance carriers have regarding infertility. Instead of regarding infertility treatment as essential as, say, obstetrical services, infertility is often considered optional, experimental, nonessential, elective. In a handful of states, laws now mandate that infertility be covered comprehensively by insurance carriers. This is terrific news, but if you don't live in one of those states, filing creatively is the only method of making sure you can recover at least some of your costs.

It's time to act as soon as you realize you may be in for a battery of tests for infertility. Even with all the emotional turmoil that may be associated with beginning a fertility investigation, try to stay alert to the cost-recovery methods you'll be using. If you have insurance, check it out thoroughly to see what is covered. Consider purchasing a separate plan if you find it is more cost-effective for infertility in the long run. You can ask independent agents (insurance agents who represent several companies) to help you seek good coverage.

Find out about old and new policies:

- What will your basic coverage pay for in terms of infertility?
- What is your deductible?
- What percentage of each fee is covered?
- How long do we wait to be reimbursed?
- Can basic coverage be boosted by purchasing more insurance?
- Will it be worth the extra payments in the long run?
- How does your coverage differ for office visits, tests, medication, surgery, OR charges, anesthesia, etc.?
- Who files: the doctor, hospital, or you? Is this always true?
- Would shopping around for a completely new policy be worthwhile?
- Is infertility counseling, if needed, covered?
- Are there laws in your state which regulate coverage of infertility costs?

Some insurance plans pay the bills directly for you, but most people must cover the costs first and wait to be reimbursed. If this is your case, be very careful that you don't lose track of any of your claims. As the receipts begin to pile up, you must keep a handle on your progress in cost recovery, and see to it yourself that your claims are moving along efficiently.

File promptly. Try to make it a rule to mail in (or be sure your doctor mails in) your claims within forty-eight hours.

- Make copies of everything! Prescriptions before you fill them, all receipts, doctor bills, filled-out claims. Before you send these documents away, be sure you have a record of them. When claims are lost or disputed, you can refer to your copies.

- Keep diagnoses consistent and as "technical" as possible. While "infertility" may not be covered, "oligospermia" could be. And in cases of IVF or GIFT procedures, breaking the process down to its component parts can help you get it covered. Ask your doctors and their assistants for advice on filing nomenclature.
- Get to know the biller at your doctor's so you can ask questions and follow up on your claims in a friendly manner.
- Do not hesitate to ask to have your forms filled out or to be given complete receipts.
- Keep your claims moving. If you have two policies that overlap, record which claim is going where.
- Check off amounts repaid to you against full original costs and see if your reimbursements are correct.
- When going into the hospital, do as much advance paperwork as you can.
- Date everything with day of service, day of payment, day you filed. Keep your paperwork in chronological order according to the filing date.

Here's a simple form that will help you keep track of your payments, what they are for, and filing information:

THE INFERTILITY MAZE

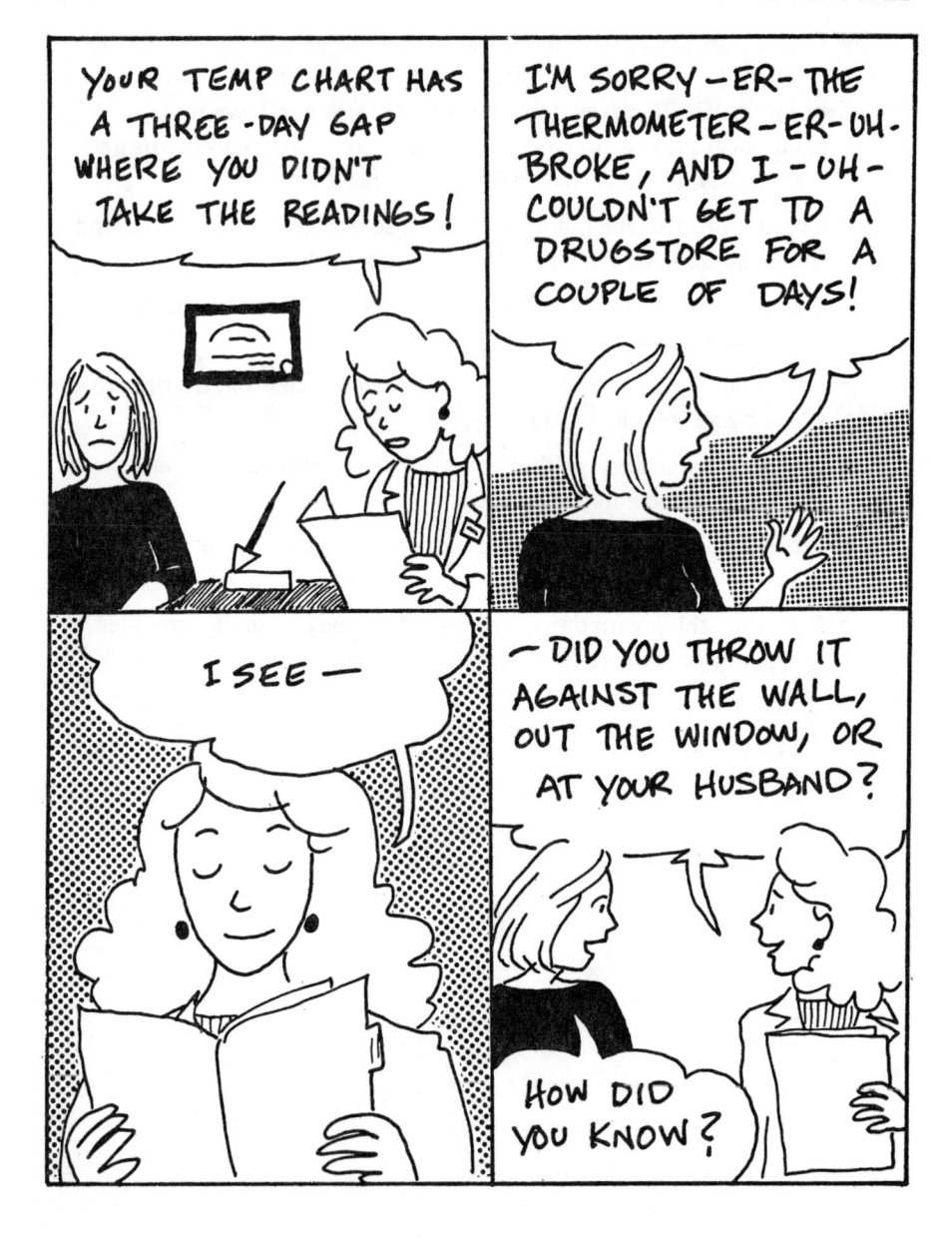

INSURANCE POLICY INFORMATION AT A GLANCE
(For filling out forms at the doctor's)

Carrier A

Company _____

Identification or Policy Numbers _____
_____

Policy in name of _____

Type of policy _____
_____

Expiration or other dated information _____

Infertility coverage _____
_____

Contact in case of mistakes: _____
_____
_____

Other information: _____
_____
_____
_____

Carrier B

Company _____

Identification or Policy Numbers _____
_____

Policy in name of _____

Type of policy _____

_____

Expiration or other dated information _____

Infertility coverage _____

_____

Contact in case of mistakes: _____

_____

_____

Other information: _____

_____

_____

_____

RECORD OF INSURANCE CLAIMS

Date of Service	Nature of Service	Doctor	Costs	Date Claim Filed	Date of Refund	Amount Refunded	Our Total Cost	Notes

RECORD OF BASAL BODY TEMPERATURE

NAME _____ CYCLE FROM: _____ TO: _____

Date	Cycle Day	Temperature	Other Information
	1	96.5 6 7 8 9 97.0 1 2 3 4 5 6 7 8 9 98.0 1 2 3 4 5 6 7 8 9 99.0	
	2	96.5 6 7 8 9 97.0 1 2 3 4 5 6 7 8 9 98.0 1 2 3 4 5 6 7 8 9 99.0	
	3	96.5 6 7 8 9 97.0 1 2 3 4 5 6 7 8 9 98.0 1 2 3 4 5 6 7 8 9 99.0	
	4	96.5 6 7 8 9 97.0 1 2 3 4 5 6 7 8 9 98.0 1 2 3 4 5 6 7 8 9 99.0	
	5	96.5 6 7 8 9 97.0 1 2 3 4 5 6 7 8 9 98.0 1 2 3 4 5 6 7 8 9 99.0	
	6	96.5 6 7 8 9 97.0 1 2 3 4 5 6 7 8 9 98.0 1 2 3 4 5 6 7 8 9 99.0	
	7	96.5 6 7 8 9 97.0 1 2 3 4 5 6 7 8 9 98.0 1 2 3 4 5 6 7 8 9 99.0	
	8	96.5 6 7 8 9 97.0 1 2 3 4 5 6 7 8 9 98.0 1 2 3 4 5 6 7 8 9 99.0	
	9	96.5 6 7 8 9 97.0 1 2 3 4 5 6 7 8 9 98.0 1 2 3 4 5 6 7 8 9 99.0	
	10	96.5 6 7 8 9 97.0 1 2 3 4 5 6 7 8 9 98.0 1 2 3 4 5 6 7 8 9 99.0	
	11	96.5 6 7 8 9 97.0 1 2 3 4 5 6 7 8 9 98.0 1 2 3 4 5 6 7 8 9 99.0	
	12	96.5 6 7 8 9 97.0 1 2 3 4 5 6 7 8 9 98.0 1 2 3 4 5 6 7 8 9 99.0	
	13	96.5 6 7 8 9 97.0 1 2 3 4 5 6 7 8 9 98.0 1 2 3 4 5 6 7 8 9 99.0	
	14	96.5 6 7 8 9 97.0 1 2 3 4 5 6 7 8 9 98.0 1 2 3 4 5 6 7 8 9 99.0	
	15	96.5 6 7 8 9 97.0 1 2 3 4 5 6 7 8 9 98.0 1 2 3 4 5 6 7 8 9 99.0	
	16	96.5 6 7 8 9 97.0 1 2 3 4 5 6 7 8 9 98.0 1 2 3 4 5 6 7 8 9 99.0	
	17	96.5 6 7 8 9 97.0 1 2 3 4 5 6 7 8 9 98.0 1 2 3 4 5 6 7 8 9 99.0	
	18	96.5 6 7 8 9 97.0 1 2 3 4 5 6 7 8 9 98.0 1 2 3 4 5 6 7 8 9 99.0	
	19	96.5 6 7 8 9 97.0 1 2 3 4 5 6 7 8 9 98.0 1 2 3 4 5 6 7 8 9 99.0	
	20	96.5 6 7 8 9 97.0 1 2 3 4 5 6 7 8 9 98.0 1 2 3 4 5 6 7 8 9 99.0	
	21	96.5 6 7 8 9 97.0 1 2 3 4 5 6 7 8 9 98.0 1 2 3 4 5 6 7 8 9 99.0	
	22	96.5 6 7 8 9 97.0 1 2 3 4 5 6 7 8 9 98.0 1 2 3 4 5 6 7 8 9 99.0	
	23	96.5 6 7 8 9 97.0 1 2 3 4 5 6 7 8 9 98.0 1 2 3 4 5 6 7 8 9 99.0	
	24	96.5 6 7 8 9 97.0 1 2 3 4 5 6 7 8 9 98.0 1 2 3 4 5 6 7 8 9 99.0	
	25	96.5 6 7 8 9 97.0 1 2 3 4 5 6 7 8 9 98.0 1 2 3 4 5 6 7 8 9 99.0	
	26	96.5 6 7 8 9 97.0 1 2 3 4 5 6 7 8 9 98.0 1 2 3 4 5 6 7 8 9 99.0	
	27	96.5 6 7 8 9 97.0 1 2 3 4 5 6 7 8 9 98.0 1 2 3 4 5 6 7 8 9 99.0	
	28	96.5 6 7 8 9 97.0 1 2 3 4 5 6 7 8 9 98.0 1 2 3 4 5 6 7 8 9 99.0	
	29	96.5 6 7 8 9 97.0 1 2 3 4 5 6 7 8 9 98.0 1 2 3 4 5 6 7 8 9 99.0	
	30	96.5 6 7 8 9 97.0 1 2 3 4 5 6 7 8 9 98.0 1 2 3 4 5 6 7 8 9 99.0	
	31	96.5 6 7 8 9 97.0 1 2 3 4 5 6 7 8 9 98.0 1 2 3 4 5 6 7 8 9 99.0	
	32	96.5 6 7 8 9 97.0 1 2 3 4 5 6 7 8 9 98.0 1 2 3 4 5 6 7 8 9 99.0	

THE ALTERNATIVES

RECORD OF BASAL BODY TEMPERATURE

NAME _____   CYCLE FROM: _____ TO: _____

Resources: Important Names and Addresses

DOCTORS, HOSPITALS, AND CLINICS

Doctor _____

Specialty _____

Address and phone _____

_____

Referred by _____

Notes: _____

_____

_____

_____

Doctor _____

Specialty _____

Address and phone _____

_____

Referred by _____

Notes: _____

_____

_____

_____

LABORATORIES

Name of lab _____

Address and phone _____

_____

Recommended by _____

Tests performed and prices _____

_____

_____

_____

_____

Name of lab _____

Address and phone _____

_____

Recommended by _____

Tests performed and prices _____

_____

_____

_____

_____

Medication Records

It is important to keep track of what medication is prescribed for you, what dosage is taken, and if the drug helped you or not. Your present doctor will want to know, and if you should consult another specialist, you will be able to accurately describe your treatment.

MEDICATION RECORD

Prescribing Doctor _____

Address and phone _____

_____

Medication _____

_____

Dosage _____

_____

_____

Prescribed for what problem? _____

_____

_____

Medication taken beginning date _____

_____

Ended medication date _____

_____

Stopped for what reason? _____

_____

_____

Improvements, side effects, changes, and dates noted: _____

_____

_____

_____

_____

_____

Costs _____

Pharmacy where obtained _____

Address and phone _____

_____

MEDICATION RECORD

Prescribing Doctor _____

Address and phone _____

Medication _____

Dosage _____

Prescribed for what problem? _____

Medication taken beginning date _____

Ended medication date _____

Stopped for what reason? _____

Improvements, side effects, changes, and dates noted: _____

Costs _____

Pharmacy where obtained _____

Address and phone _____

MEDICATION RECORD

Prescribing Doctor _____

Address and phone _____

Medication _____

Dosage _____

Prescribed for what problem? _____

Medication taken beginning date _____

Ended medication date _____

Stopped for what reason? _____

Improvements, side effects, changes, and dates noted: _____

_____

_____

_____

_____

Costs _____

Pharmacy where obtained _____

Address and phone _____

MEDICATION RECORD

Prescribing Doctor _____

Address and phone _____

_____

Medication _____

_____

Dosage _____

_____

_____

Prescribed for what problem? _____

_____

_____

Medication taken beginning date _____

_____

Ended medication date _____

_____

Stopped for what reason? _____

_____

_____

_____

Improvements, side effects, changes, and dates noted: _____

_____

_____

_____

_____

Costs _____

Pharmacy where obtained _____

Address and phone _____

_____

Bibliography

Books

Andrews, Lori. *New Conceptions.* New York: Ballantine Books, 1985.

Bellina, Joseph, M.D., Ph.D., and Wilson, Josleen. *You Can Have a Baby.* New York: Bantam Books, 1986.

Berg, Barbara. *Nothing to Cry About.* New York: Seaview Books, 1981.

Bolles, Edmund B. *The Penguin Adoption Handbook.* New York: Penguin Books, 1984.

Bombardieri, Merle. *The Baby Decision.* New York: Rawson-Wade Publishers, 1981.

Corea, Gena. *The Mother Machine.* New York: Harper & Row, 1985.

Faux, Marilyn. *Childless by Choice.* New York: Anchor Press, 1984.

Gilman, Lois. *The Adoption Resource Book.* New York: Harper & Row, 1984.

Glass, Robert H., and Ericsson, Ronald J. *Getting Pregnant in the 1980s.* Berkeley: University of California Press, 1982.

Hammond, Mary, M.D., and Talbot, Luther, M.D. *Infertility: A Practical Guide for the Physician.* Oradell, N.J.: Medical Economics Books, 1985.

Johnston, Patricia I. *An Adoptor's Advocate.* Fort Wayne, Ind.: Perspectives Press, 1984.

———. *Understanding: A Guide to Impaired Fertility for Family and Friends.* Fort Wayne, Ind.: Perspectives Press, 1983.

Kushner, Harold. *When Bad Things Happen to Good People.* New York: Schocken Books, 1981.

Mazor, Miriam. *Infertility: Medical, Emotional, and Social Considerations.* New York: Human Sciences Press, 1984.

Mennings, Barbara Eck. *Infertility: A Guide for the Childless Couple.* New York: Prentice Hall Press, 1977.

Older, Julia. *Endometriosis.* New York: Charles Scribner's Sons, 1984.

Perloe, Mark, M.D., and Christine, Linda Gail. *Miracle Babies and Other Happy Endings.* New York: Rawson Associates, 1986.

Pfeiffer, Regina A., and Whitlock, Katherine. *Fertility Awareness.* New York: Prentice-Hall Press, 1984.

Pizer, Hank, and O'Brien, Christine. *Coping with a Miscarriage.* New York: Dial Press, 1980.

Salzer, Linda. *Infertility: How Couples Can Cope.* Boston: G. K. Hall, 1986.

Silber, Sherman, M.D. *How to Get Pregnant.* New York: Warner Books, 1980.

Tilton, Nan, Tilton, Todd, and Moore, Gaylen. *Making Miracles.* New York: Doubleday, 1985.

Whelen, Elizabeth. *A Baby: Maybe.* New York: Bobbs-Merrill, 1975.

Articles, Monographs, Pamphlets, Fact Sheets

Bombardieri, Merle. "Childfree Decision-Making." RESOLVE fact sheet, © RESOLVE, Inc.

Brozan, Nadine. "Rising Use of Donated Eggs for Pregnancy Stirs Concern." *New York Times,* January 18, 1988, p. A1.

Burns, Linda Hammer. "Effective Decision-Making." *Perspectives on Infertility,* vol. 4, no. 1, January-February 1986, pp. 3-5.

"Causes and Treatment of Male Infertility." *Perspectives on Infertility,* vol. 2, no. 4, March-April 1984, pp. 4-11.

Chase, Anne. "Want-Ad Babies." *The Washingtonian,* August 1987, pp, 102-7, 152-59.

Corman, Carolyn. "Trying (And Trying and Trying) To Get Pregnant." *Ms.,* May 1983, pp. 21-24.

Davis, Gwen. "The Private Pain of Infertility." *New York Times Magazine,* December 6, 1987, pp. 106-21.

DeBrovner, Charles, M.D. "The Infertility Workup." *Perspectives on Infertility.* vol. 3, no. 6, November-December 1985, pp. 3-8.

DES Action National. "DES Exposure: Questions and Answers." Long Island Jewish Hospital, New Hyde Park, N.Y. 10040. (pamphlet)

Dubin, Lawrence, M.D., and Amelar, Richard, M.D. "Varicocele," *Urologic Clinics of North America,* vol. 5, no. 3, October 1978. (reprint)

Eagen, Andra B. "Baby Roulette." *The Village Voice,* August 25, 1987, pp. 17-21.

Elliott, Laura. "At Last, a Baby." *The Washingtonian,* January 1988, pp. 108-23.

Fleming, Jeanne, Ph.D. "Infertility as a Chronic Illness." RESOLVE Fact Sheet, © RESOLVE, Inc.

Harris, Diane. "What It Costs to Fight Infertility." *Money,* December 1984, pp. 201-12.

"Infertility: A Growing Array of Remedies." *New York Times,* February 11, 1986, p. c12.

"Infertility: New Cures, New Hope." *Newsweek,* December 6, 1982, pp. 102-10.

"Insurers Refusing to Pay Some Costs in Infertility Cases." *New York Times,* February 10, 1986, p. B7.

Jacoby, Susan. "The Baby Bandwagon." *Glamour,* September 1987, pp. 388-90, 430-32.

Kantrow, Barbara, et al. "Who Keeps Baby M?" *Newsweek,* January 19, 1987, pp. 44-51.

Kramer, Michael. "Last Chance Babies." *New York,* August 12, 1985, pp. 134-42.

Levine, Judith. "Whose Baby Is It?" *The Village Voice,* November 25, 1986, pp. 15-22.

Lewis, Susan. "The Emotional Impact of Infertility." *Glamour,* December 1985, pp. 244-46, 288-91.

Lord, Lewis J., et al. "Desperately Seeking Baby." *US News and World Report,* October 5, 1987, pp. 58-65.

Mahlstedt, Patricia, Ed.D. "The Psychological Component of Infertility." *Fertility and Sterility,* vol. 43, no. 3, March 1985, pp. 335-45.

Menning, Barbara Eck. "Counseling Infertile Couples." Reprint from *OB/GYN,* February 1979, ©RESOLVE, Inc.

———. "The Emotional Needs of Infertile Couples," *Fertility and Sterility,* vol. 34, no. 4, October 1980, pp. 313-19.

Pogash, Carol. "This Story Has a Happy Ending." *Redbook,* August 1982, pp. 81-86.

Randal, Judith E. "A Laser Alternative to the D & C." *New York Newsday,* December 29, 1987, p. D9.

"Overview of Adoption." RESOLVE, Inc. Fact Sheet. ©RESOLVE, Inc.

Rosenberg, Jane. "Taking an Active Role in Resolving Infertility." *Perspectives in Infertility,* January-February 1986, pp. 12-14.

Rosenthal, Miriam B., M.D. "Grappling With the Emotional Aspects of Infertility." *Contemporary OB/GYN,* July 1985, pp. 97-105.

Seligmann, Jean, et al. "The Grueling Baby Chase." *Newsweek,* November 30, 1987, pp. 78-82.

Shubin, Roselle. "Artificial Insemination." *Perspectives on Infertility,* January-February, pp. 12-14.

"Vatican Seeks Curb on Birth Technology." *New York Times,* March 11, 1987, pp. A1, B14-17.

White, Ralph de Vere, M.D. "Medical Management of Male Infertility." RESOLVE Fact Sheet, ©RESOLVE, Inc.

Index

Abortions, and incidence of infertility, 12–13
Achievement anxiety, and infertility, 17
Acquisitiveness, and infertility, 17
Adoption, 19, 225–34, 244–45
  facts about, 231–32
  getting information on, 227, 248–49
  questions concerning, 225–27
  and spontaneous pregnancy, 22–23
  types of, 228–30
Age, relationship of, to fertility, 9
Agency adoption, 228–29
AID. *See* Artificial insemination, donor (AID)
AIH. *See* Artificial insemination, homologous (AIH, IAIH)
Alternatives, 200–201. *See also* Treatment
  adoption as, 225–34, 244–45
  artificial insemination, donor (AID), 207–13
  childfree living, 235–41, 242–43
  egg donation, 219–20
  embryo freezing, 220
  embryo transfer, 219
  and the need to grieve, 203–5
  sperm donation, 220
  surrogate parenting, 215–18
  talking about, 201–3
American Fertility Society, 28, 161, 247
Amniocentesis, 191
Andrologist, 26
Artificial insemination, 19, 20
Artificial insemination, donor (AID), 207–13
  emotional considerations, 208–9
  and issue of secrecy, 209–10
  legal paperwork in, 212
  practical considerations, 209–12

  process of, 212–13
  screening of donors, 211
  using fresh or frozen sperm, 211–12
Artificial insemination, homologous (AIH, IAIH), 167, 168, 181, 182–85, 208
  considerations in, 183
  definition of, 182–83
  process of, 184–85
Asherman's syndrome, 173
Azodspermia, 103, 104, 214

Balloon method of treating varicocele, 178–79
Basal body temperature (BBT), 38–39
  charts for keeping, 38–39, 256–57
  interpreting charts, 69–70, 73–74
  taking and recording, 40–42
  thoughts on taking, 43
Beta-HCG test, 173
Biological clock, 9
Birth control usage, and incidence of infertility, 12
Blood testing
  to check female hormonal level, 70
  to check male hormonal level, 111
  and miscarriage, 172
  to track ovulation, 69, 70
Bombardieri, Merle, 136
Boxer shorts, and infertility, 32
Bradshaw, Judy, 197
Bromocriptine
  to treat male hormonal problems, 180
  to treat ovulation problems, 159

Calendar, sexual relations by, 46–47
CAT-scan, 98
Cervix/cervical mucus
  condition of, 77–78

examination of, in postcoital test, 71–72
and miscarriage, 172
treatment for problems with, 166–67
watching for changes in, 45–46
Childfree living, 235–43
getting information on, 249
Chlamydia, 111
Clomid, 19
to treat luteal phase defect, 160
to treat male hormonal problems, 180
to treat ovulation problems, 151–54, 167
to treat varicocele, 179
Clomiphene citrate
to treat male hormonal problems, 180
to treat ovulation problems, 151–54
Clumping, 112
Colposcope, 169
Communication, and infertility, 136–39
Corpus luteum, 39
Cortisone therapy, for male hormonal problems, 180–81
Cough syrup, use of, as home remedy, 32
Counseling
and acceptance of infertility diagnosis, 119–20
need for, 149–50

Danazol, to treat endometriosis, 162–63
Danocrine, to treat endometriosis, 162–63
DES Action National, 169, 247
DES (diethylstilbestrol) exposure
and incidence of infertility, 13
getting information on, 247–48
and miscarriage, 172
treatment for problems with, 166–70

Diagnostic laparoscopy. *See* Laparoscopy
Drugs, and incidence of infertility, 13–14
Dueckman, Amy, 78–81, 87–90

Ectopic pregnancy, 173
Egg donation, 219–20
Embryo freezing, 220
Embryo transfer, 219
Endometrial biopsy, 19, 69, 70, 79, 173
aftereffects of, 87
procedure in, 84–85, 87
record of, 86
Endometriosis, 88
confirmation of diagnosis of, 161
getting information on, 248
and incidence of infertility, 12
and miscarriage, 172
treatments for, 161–62
Danazol, 162–63
GnRH analogue, 163
surgery, 163–64
Endometriosis Association, 161, 248
Environmental factors
and incidence of infertility, 14
and miscarriage, 172

Fallopian tubes, treating problems with, 164–65
Ferning, 72
Fertility, relationship of, to age, 9
Fimbria, 89
Fleming, Dr. Jeanne, 122
FSH (follicle-stimulating hormone), and basal body temperature, 38–39

George, Katie, 132–33, 223
Gerety, Margie, 196
GIFT (gamete intre-fallopian transfer), 167, 168, 185, 191–92, 208
preparing for, 193

INDEX 269

and use of Pergonal, 155
GnRH (gonadotropin-releasing hormone)
  to treat endometriosis, 163–64
  to treat ovulation problems, 159
Grief, need for, 117, 203–5, 226

Hagerty, Dorothy, 19–20, 43
Hamster test, 112
Harris, Lisa, 145
HCG. *See* Human Chorionic Gonadotropin (HCG)
HMG. *See* Human Menopausal Gonadotropin (HMG)
Health-maintenance organizations (HMO), and coverage of in vitro fertilization, 187
Hormones
  blood work for detecting levels of
    in men, 111
    in women, 70, 74
How to Get Pregnant (Silbur), 11
Hudson, Jeffrey, 108–109
Human Chorionic Gonadotropin (HCG)
  to treat luteal phase defect, 160
  to treat male hormonal problems, 180
  to treat varicocele, 179
Human Menopausal Gonadotropin (HMG)
  use of, in treating ovulation problems, 155–58
Hyperprolactinemia, 180
Hysterosalpingogram, 19, 79–81, 165, 169, 173
  aftereffects, 83
  procedure in, 83
  record of, 82
Hysteroscopy, 97

IAIH. *See* Artificial insemination, homologous (AIH, IAIH)
Identified adoption, 229–30
Immunity problems, treatment of, 168
Impatience, and infertility, 17
Incompetent cervix, 167
Independent adoption, 229–30
Infections, and infertility, 167
Infertility
  accepting, 214
  anxiety concerning, 9–17
  definition of, 10
  emotional impact of, 1, 4, 132–33
  in everyday living, 129–31
  getting information about, 29–31, 246–49
  home remedies for, 31–33
  impact of, 19–20, 21
  importance of communication in resolving, 4–5
  investigating causes of, 5
  methods of coping with, 67
  need for knowledge concerning, 3–4
  need for second opinion, 121
  negative diagnosis of, 120–23
  philosophical and religious considerations in, 142–44
  positive diagnosis of, 117–20
  pregnancy after, 194–98
  resolving, 1–2
  statistics on incidence of, 11–12
  treatment of, as secret, 140–44
Infertility clinics, 26–27
Infertility maze, 1–6
Infertility workup
  coping with inconveniences of, 63–67
  emotional impact of, 51–52
  evaluation of specialist, 53–55
  insurance coverage for, 66–67
  for men, 62–63
    bloodwork, 111
    invasive tests, 112–113
    physical exam, 110–111
    semen analysis, 99–107
    sperm testing, 111–112
  planning of, 57–59
  questions for first appointment, 55–56

talking with doctor concerning,
    56–57
for women, 59–61
    CAT-scan, 98
    endometrial biopsy, 84–87
    hysterosalpingogram, 79–83
    hysteroscopy, 97
    karyotyping, 99
    laparoscopy, 88–91, 93–96
    notes on, 73–76
    physical and pelvic exam, 68–69
    postcoital test, 71–72, 77–78
    radiology work, 97–98
    tracking ovulation, 69–70
    ultrasound, 98–99
Insurance and cost recovery, 249–55
    and GnRH treatment, 159
    and in vitro fertilization, 187
International adoption, 229
In vitro fertilization (IVF), 19, 167,
    168, 185–91
    emotional considerations, 188–89
    ethical considerations, 189
    insurance coverage for, 187
    practical considerations, 186–87
    process of, 189–91
    and use of Pergonal, 155

Johnson, Margaret, 185, 242
Johnston, Patricia I., 138

Karyotyping, 99
Kubler-Ross, Elisabeth, 117

Laparoscopy, 19, 88–90, 173
    preparing for, 93
    procedure in, 93–99
    record of, 91
LH (luteinizing hormone), and the
    basal body temperature, 38–39
Luteal phase defect, treatment for,
    159–60

Manzo, Jean Quinn, 170
Marijuana, and incidence of
    infertility, 14

Mason, Mary, 233–34
Medical history, reviewing, 33–37
Medication records, 259–63
Men
    infertility workup for, 62–63
        bloodwork, 111
        invasive tests, 112–113
        physical exam, 110–111
        semen analysis, 99–107
        sperm testing, 111–112
    treatment of infertility in,
        blockage of sperm ducts, 181
        hormonal problems, 179–81
        seminal fluid problems, 181–82
        varicocele, 177–79
Menning, Barbara Eck, 117, 122, 204
Menstrual cycle
    impact of stress on, 21
    irregularity of, 12
Milford, Jennifer, 193
Miscarriage, 171–77
    actions to take in case of, 174–75
    clues to infertility related, 172–73
    and ectopic pregnancy, 173
Missionary position, 32
Mittelschmerz, 45–46, 133
Motrin, 79–80
Multiple births, and use of Pergonal,
    156
Mumps, and incidence of infertility,
    13
Mycoplasm, 111
Myomectomy, 197

National Adoption Exchange, 249
Natural conception, timing of, 10
North American Council on
    Adoptable Children, 249

Obstetrician-gynecologist, 24
    as infertility specialist, 24–25
Oligospermia, 103, 208
Orgasm, and infertility, 32–33
Orphan embryos, 220
OURS, Inc., 248

INDEX

Ovulation
  tracking of, for infertility workup, 44-45, 69-70, 73-74
  treatment for problems in
    clomiphene citrate, 151-54
    GnRH (gonadotropin-releasing hormone), 159
    Human Menopausal Gonadotropin, 155-58
    parlodel, 159

Pap smear, 68
Parlodel
  to treat male hormonal problems, 180
  to treat ovulation problems, 159
Pelvic exam, in infertility workup, 68-69, 73
Pelvic infections, and incidence of infertility, 12
Pelvic inflammatory disease, 171
  and incidence of infertility, 12
Penetrak test, 112
Penis, checking of, in infertility workup, 110
Pergonal, to treat ovulation problems, 155-58
Peters, Carol, 140-44
Physical
  in infertility workup
    for men, 110-11
    for women, 68-69, 73
Postcoital test, 71-72
  emotional impact of having, 77-78
  preparing for, 78
  record of, 75-76
Pregnancy
  after infertility, 194-98
  handling of, in friend, 142
  phenomenon of spontaneous, 22-23
Pregnancy and Infant Loss Center, 248
Private adoption, 229-30

Radiology work, 97-98

Reproductive endocrinology/ infertility, specialist in, 25
RESOLVE, Inc., 6, 17-18, 28, 31, 117, 119
  getting counseling through, 119, 150
  getting information from, 125, 143, 152, 160, 246
  getting referral through, 121
Resources
  laboratories, 259
  names and addresses, 258
Ross, Mary Shields, 145
Rubin's insufflation test, 79

Schwan, Kassie, 93-99
Scrotal cooling, to treat varicocele, 177-78
Semen analysis, 19, 32, 72, 99-107
  agglutination, 104
  azodspermia, 103, 104
  liquefaction, 102
  morphology, 103
  motility, 102-3
  sperm count, 103-104
  viscosity, 102
  volume, 102
Seminal fluid, treatment for problems with, 181-82
Serophene
  to treat male hormonal problems, 180
  to treat ovulation problems, 151-54
Sexually transmitted diseases, and infertility, 12, 13, 167
Sexual relations
  by the calendar, 46-47
  timing of, 33
Silber, Dr. Sherman, 11
Sims-Huhner test. *See* Postcoital test
Smoking, and incidence of infertility, 13-14
Specialist
  finding and choosing, 27-29
  need for, 23-24

types of, 24–27
Special need kids, adoption of, 230–31
Speculum, 68
Sperm count, 72, 103–104
Sperm donation, 220
Sperm duct blockage, surgical repair of, 181
Sperm washing, 223
Stress, impact of, on menstrual cycle, 21
Support groups, 148–49
Surgery
  for endometriosis, 163–64
  for sperm duct blockage, 181
Surrogate parenting, 215–18

Temperature. *See* Basal body temperature (BBT)
Testicle, undescended, and incidence of infertility, 13
Testicular biopsy, 112–13
Testosterone, for male hormonal problems, 181
Thelen, Lisa Giblin, 77–78
Thermometers, types of, 39
Treatment
  for both partners
    artificial insemination, homologous (AIH, IAIH), 182–85
    GIFT (gamete intre-fallopian transfer), 191–92
    in vitro fertilization (IVF), 185–91
  deciding to end, 221–25
  for men
    blockage of sperm ducts, 181
    hormonal problems, 179–81
    seminal fluid problems, 181–82
    varicocele, 177–79
  need for support groups, 148–49
  planning of, 123–24
  questions concerning proposed, 124–25

questions to answer concerning surgery, 126–27
reassessing, 127–29
religious restrictions on, 144
taking a break in, 146–48
use of counseling in, 149–51
for women
  cervix/cervical mucus, 166–67
  DES exposure, 168–70
  endometriosis, 161–64
  fallopian tube defects, 164–65
  immunity problems, 168
  for luteal phase defect, 159–60
  miscarriage as special problem, 171–77
  ovulation problems, 151–59
  pelvic inflammatory disease, 171
  uterine problems, 165–66
"Twenty-Minute Rule," 136, 137

Ultrasound, 98–99
  to track ovulation, 70
  and use of Pergonal, 155–56
Understanding—A Guide to Impaired Fertility for Family and Friends (Johnston), 138
Ureaplasma, 111
  and miscarriage, 172
Urine testing, to track ovulation, 69
Urine testing kits, 44–45
Urologist, 26, 110
Uterine problems, treatment of, 165–66

Varicocele, 110–111
  treatment of, 177–79
Vasogram, 112–113
  to repair sperm duct blockage, 181

Waiting children, adoption of, 230–31
Webster, Bonnie, 206
Women
  infertility workup for, 59–61
    CAT-scan, 98
    endometrial biopsy, 84–87

hysterosalpinogram, 79–83
  hysteroscopy, 97
  karyotyping, 99
  laparoscopy, 88–91, 93–96
  notes on, 73–76
  physical and pelvic exam, 68–69
  post-coital test, 71–72, 77–78
  radiology work, 97–98
  tracking ovulation, 69–70
  ultrasound, 98–99
 treatment of infertility in
  cervix/cervical mucus, 166–67
  DES exposure, 168–70
  endometriosis, 161–64
  fallopian tube defects, 164–65
  immunity problems, 168
  for luteal phase defect, 159–60
  miscarriage as special problem, 171–77
  ovulation problems, 151–59
  pelvic inflammatory disease, 171
  uterine problems, 165–66
Wusinich, Denise, 83–85